MILLIONS OF AMERICAN WOMEN HAVE SHARED A COMMON EXPERIENCE

We have used and trusted tampons.

We believed that they were safe, medically tested and approved.

We never dreamed that a tiny wad of fiber may contribute to serious illness or injury.

We found out that we were wrong.

EVERYTHING YOU MUST KNOW ABOUT TAMPONS

Nancy Friedman

With An Introduction by
Cynthia W. Cooke, M.D.

BERKLEY BOOKS, NEW YORK

Grateful acknowledgment is offered to the following:

Johnson & Johnson, Inc. for permission to reproduce the anatomical drawing from the o.b. package insert;

Tampax, Inc. for permission to reproduce an advertisement;

Personal Products Company for permission to reproduce the Meds advertisement;

Purex Industries, Inc. for permission to reproduce the Pursettes advertisement;

Obstetrics and Gynecology for permission to reproduce an anatomical drawing of the menstrual cup in place;

John Wiley & Sons, Inc. for permission to reproduce an anatomical drawing from BIOLOGY OF WOMEN, by Ethel Sloane, copyright © 1980 by John Wiley & Sons, Inc.

EVERYTHING YOU MUST KNOW
ABOUT TAMPONS

A Berkley Book / published by arrangement with
the author

PRINTING HISTORY
Berkley edition / June 1981

ISBN: 0-425-05140-4

A BERKLEY BOOK® TM 757,375

PRINTED IN THE UNITED STATES OF AMERICA

Acknowledgments

A great many people helped me with my research. Rosalie Muller Wright, Jon Carroll and especially B.K. Moran, my editor for the original article, earned my deepest gratitude for believing in me from the start and fighting to get the information published. Many women's self-care clinics around the country cooperated with my survey and answered questions about tampon use among their patients. Sandra E. Ritz was an inspiration, an invaluable source of information and a friend. Dr. Dean Edell of San Francisco's KGO radio and TV was most gracious about sharing the important consumer feedback he received. Peat O'Neil and Charlotte Oram of Woman Health International saved me hours of time with their comprehensive bibliography and review of medical literature on tampons. I was blessed with a research assistant, Nan Silver, and an editor, Linda Healey, who were both knowledgeable and caring. Finally, I want to thank Jim and Matt Cord for tolerating and loving me during almost two years of tampon research. As they'll attest, it wasn't always easy.

Contents

Introduction

by *Cynthia W. Cooke, M.D.*
Assistant Clinical Professor
Obstetrics and Gynecology
University of Pennsylvania

The nightmare of Toxic Shock Syndrome (TSS) came upon us in the last two years, catching women and their doctors unawares. A new disease, especially an infectious one, is always startling. But TSS was especially bothersome for two reasons: it was killing previously healthy young women, and it seemed to be associated with widely-used products which had been considered innocuous. This assumption of safety was not justified. Ms. Friedman lucidly shows us in her detailed review of the medical literature that though TSS is the most severe problem to be associated with tampon use, many other complaints and disorders have been reported over the years. These reports have been given little attention by the medical community, the lay press or the regulatory agencies. In fact, the tampon manufacturers were drastically changing the composition of their devices over the past decade without a whimper from anyone but a few women's groups until the TSS disaster.

In my gynecologic practice I have seen numbers of women over the past few years who have had problems which I now believe to have been associated with tampon usage—chronic recurrent vaginitis and a strange laceration at the top of one woman's vagina. Several of my patients have had vaginal ulcers which rapidly cleared after discontinuing tampon use. Two other women were interesting in the similarity of their stories and symptoms. Both gave the history of daily bleeding for over a year. On careful questioning, their tampon use was astounding. Each had worn a tampon every day since the bleeding had begun. The bleeding was scant except for the time of their periods when they would change tampons several times daily. Otherwise, they would leave a tampon in place for twenty-four hours, remove it in the morning and if there was any blood present (there always was), insert another. Needless to say, by the time I examined them, each had significant excoriation and ulceration of the upper vagina. The ulcers healed rapidly and the bleeding stopped after discontinuing tampon use. Clearly, both the product and the user were involved in these cases.

In this regard, it has continued to astonish me that so many women use tampons between periods. Societal taboos, fanned by the pressures of Madison Avenue advertising agencies, have convinced many women that all vaginal drainage, be it blood or normal mucus, is dirty, something to be hidden or dammed up. Along this line, I must offer a speculation, which is shared by some of my medical colleagues. Could it be that the severe menstrual cramps that some women experience while using tampons may be due to retrograde menstruation? That is, do the tampons so effectively block the outlet to the vagina that the blood flows back through the Fallopian tubes and into the abdominal cavity? This was one of the theories expounded in trying to explain the mechanism of TSS. It remains entirely theoretical but worrisome nonetheless. If one day this mechanism is conclusively demonstrated, we may also have an explanation for the apparent increase in the prevalence of endometriosis over the last few decades. In this condition, the normal lining tissue of the uterus, the endometrium, is found in other parts of the abdomen, and is responsible for severe menstrual cramps, abdominal pain and pain during intercourse. The sites where endometriosis most usually occurs are the posterior cul de sac (an area behind the uterus) and the ovaries. Interestingly, these are the sites where endometrial tissue would usually fall if retrograde menstruation were occurring. At present, the cause of endometriosis is unknown, but retrograde menstruation is high on most researchers' lists of possibilities. It will be interesting to follow this subject in the next decade. I know of no research which has examined this possible association of tampon use and endometriosis.

While we are awaiting new information on tampons, this book provides sound advice on safe use. The need for this advice underscores the dilemma which TSS presented to most women. They are worried about the disease, but it is quite clear that most women will not discontinue the use of tampons. Over the past decades their use has been equated with liberation and freedom, and this will not change overnight. However, the alternatives to the standard, commercial products are being used by increasing numbers of women, and many more will wish to experiment with these methods in the future.

The chapter describing the regulatory system, which allegedly protects us from dangerous drugs and devices, is most revealing. In this detailed account, Ms. Friedman shows how tampons fell into several regulatory crevices, thereby allowing companies the freedom to change the composition of their products significantly without submitting premarketing safety information normally required for "new" products. This review also shows that the post-marketing surveillance of these devices by the regulatory agencies has been essentially non-existent. Sadly, there seems to be little hope for a quick solution to the tampon problem, for the bureaucrats are now arguing about categorization and may do so for some time to come.

If we take nothing else from this book, it should be the overwhelming conclusion that we cannot rely on others to protect us from commercial products. Tampons are only one of thousands of products we will put into or onto our bodies during a lifetime. The scare of TSS should serve as a stimulus to making more informed decisions about the use of these products. Complete product labeling of ingredients is an absolute prerequisite for making these decisions and we should demand this on all products.

Doctors and consumers alike should be more active in reporting apparent bad reactions to drugs or devices to the FDA and the manufacturer. I feel somewhat guilty in not having reported the tampon-related ulcers that I had diagnosed. The fact that I have seen four or five cases suggests that this is a wide-spread problem, far greater than the relatively few reports in the medical literature suggest. If all of us had made appropriate reports, the suspicions about the changes in product composition might have arisen earlier.

Finally, we must assume that drug and device companies, while highly motivated to make money by enticing customers with glorious promises, would nonetheless prefer to sell a safe product. We must also assume that the FDA and other regulatory agencies would prefer to do a good job in protecting the citizens. We must also assume that these organizations need to be prodded with unending vigilance.

Cynthia W. Cooke

Preface

Like millions of American women, I used to take tampons for granted. They were small enough and when inserted, certainly hidden enough, to be practically ignored. When I began using them in college I was grateful, after seven years of belts and pads, to at last be free of my "diaper" and all the restrictions it imposed.

The only times tampons became a problem were when my supply ran out (particularly annoying when I happened to be traveling) or when the plumbing backed up (somehow a tampon was always the culprit.)

That there might be other reasons to be concerned about tampons didn't cross my mind until 1978. I was in the waiting room of the Berkeley Women's Health Collective, leafing through some health literature, when my eye was caught by a mimeographed sheet. "The Dangers of Tampons, or Only Women Bleed," it was titled. And it got right to the point. "Simple, convenient, hygienic and safe?" the writers asked. "Let's take a closer look." Tampons, they went on to say, weren't sterile surgical cotton as most of us had assumed. They were made of cotton and rayon fibers and chemicals that were waterproofed, bleached, lubricated and perfumed. Moreover, the Berkeley women cautioned, "there may be more. . . . The manufacturers have so far ignored repeated requests for a list of all substances contained in each brand of tampon." As for the hazards of all these unknown substances, the Berkeley group was grim: "Shreds of fibers come off inside you. . . . Tampons prevent drainage of discharge. . . . 'Super absorbent' really can dry you up too much. . . . Some women report they bleed more when using tampons."

I had to admit it was pretty startling. But not nearly as startling as another mimeographed sheet, this one posted at the receptionist's table in the health collective. There I read that tampons were suspected of containing asbestos—the same substance that has been linked to cancer among industrial workers who were exposed to it on the job site.

Now, *that* story sounded a little too far-fetched to be credible. (In fact, I've found no evidence to support it, and no test performed on tampons to date has demonstrated the presence of asbestos.) But it made me start thinking seriously about tampons, and I actually examined them for the first time. Some brands seemed to use sharp, shiny fibers—could this be the material that was suspected of being asbestos? Other tampons were perfumed so heavily that I didn't dare insert them for fear of an allergic reaction (like many people, I'm sensitive to some fragrances). The idea that I was inserting unknown and possible dangerous substances into my body each month was deeply disturbing and angering. I decided to do my own research into tampons to find out what doctors, government officials, manufacturers, women's self-care groups and individual women thought, knew or thought they knew about tampons. As it turned out, no one knew very much at all, and those who *did* know—the manufacturers—refused to divulge anything but the most generic information. That was even more disturbing. But most disturbing of all was the catalog of injuries and illnesses—tampon damage, I called it—that I learned had been associated with tampons, almost all within the last five years.

Midway through my research, the need to know suddenly became more acute. In May 1980, a newly discovered disease, toxic shock syndrome (TSS), changed our views about tampons and, indeed, about menstruation itself. I gathered all the information I'd been able to unearth and published a magazine article on tampon safety.*

The response to the article was a revelation. Thousands of women, it turned out—and dozens of doctors—apparently had had no idea of what was contained in tampons and what effects tampons were capable of causing. "I thought my body had changed, and that's why tampons were suddenly so uncomfortable," I heard again and again. "I never imagined that the *tampons* were different." I received phone calls, letters and requests to speak on the radio. Doctors, researchers and attorneys (who had now joined in because dozens of TSS victims were suing tampon companies) thanked me for providing them with the only information they'd ever read about tampons. Others offered information I'd previously been unaware of. Toxic shock syndrome, it seemed, was a catalyst that encouraged women to talk candidly—perhaps for the first time in their lives— about a function and a product that in the past had always been shrouded in privacy.

I wanted to be able to reach more women and health professionals with the important news about tampons, and this book is the result of that desire. It's not, I want to emphasize, an attempt to frighten women. Certainly the barrage of stories about toxic shock syndrome accomplished that task more than adequately. And I don't want women to jump to the conclusion that they should immediately throw away their tampons. That's unrealistic. I do believe that women have a right to know everything there is to know about a product they use regularly in an intimate and sen-

---

*"The Truth About Tampons," *New West* (October 20, 1980).

sitive part of their bodies—and thus be able to make their own informed decisions. I feel strongly that tampon manufacturers and the federal government have been seriously remiss in accepting the veil of "proprietary protection" and refusing to allow women to know exactly what it is they're inserting into their vaginas. I do believe, however, that the attitude is changing—slowly. And I feel that it's a great tragedy that it took a sometimes fatal disease to effect that change.

EVERYTHING YOU MUST KNOW ABOUT TAMPONS

CHAPTER 1

The Trouble with Tampons

Martha has chronic vaginal yeast infections—itching and discharge that never seem to go away. One month, while she's on a camping trip, Martha's menstrual period starts and she realizes she has no tampons with her. She borrows some sanitary napkins from a friend. The next month her yeast infections seem miraculously to have disappeared. When she switches back to tampons, the yeast returns.

Adrienne has to be rushed to the hospital emergency room because she is bleeding heavily from her vagina. The blood is bright red, not at all like menstrual fluid. Adrienne's doctor discovers that the bleeding originates not in her uterus but from a cut high up in her vagina—a cut, the doctor says, that could have been caused by a plastic tampon inserter.

Leslie goes to her gynecologist for a routine annual exam. While her feet are in the stirrups, her doctor makes an alarming discovery: several angry-looking sores inside Leslie's vagina. The doctor deduces a possible cause: pressure from tampons on vaginal tissue. Sure enough, when Leslie

1

stops wearing tampons, the ulcers heal by themselves. Her doctor is unable to explain how tampons caused the ulcers— or what might have happened if Leslie had continued to wear tampons.

On the third day of Rachel's menstrual period, she suddenly begins feeling nauseous. Before she has time to consider what might be the matter, her body is racked by violent diarrhea. Her temperature shoots up to 103 degrees, and she alternately burns and shakes with chills. Within an hour, she is so weak that she has to be taken to the nearest emergency room. Her blood pressure is dangerously low, and she appears to be going into shock. Fortunately, a doctor on duty recognizes her symptoms as those of Toxic Shock Syndrome (TSS), a newly identified, relatively rare, yet serious disease. A possible factor in TSS: tampons.

All of these stories are composites, but they're based on documented experiences. And they all share a common element: Each woman was a tampon user. Each woman believed that tampons were a safe, innocuous product designed and tested by scientists and approved by doctors. None of them dreamed that a tampon—just a little wad of fiber, after all—could be responsible for serious illness or injury.

Yet tampons are being implicated in an increasingly wide range of conditions, from minor irritation to—in at least one case—life-threatening hemorrhages. In many cases it's difficult to prove that tampons are the cause. The only evidence we have to go on is the fact that the illness or injury goes away when the woman stops using tampons.

The Food and Drug Administration's Bureau of Medical Devices, which is responsible for keeping an eye on the manufacture of tampons, maintains computer files of consumer and physician complaints called the Device Experience Network (DEN). As of February 1981, there were 590 complaints about tampons in the DEN—the majority filed by doctors. Many complaints concerned apparent or diagnosed cases of toxic shock syndrome. But a large number reported other kinds of problems—tampons that break apart inside the vagina, rashes and other irritations associated with the fragrance in "deodorant" tampons, ulcerations, lacerations. In some cases, physicians reported multiple cases; one doctor noted seeing 27 cases of vaginal ulcerations associated with tampon use in just two months.

In interviews and in responses to an informal survey I conducted, I learned that the DEN reports were not anomalous. Here are some of the things women told me about tampons:

"I've always used the same brand. But recently, they've been much harder to pull out. I assumed my body was changing—I'm 34. But now I'm beginning to think the tampons simply dry me out too much."

"My menstrual cramps are much worse when I use tampons than when I use sanitary napkins."

"I went to my doctor to clear up a bad case of vaginitis. He discovered that the infection was caused by the sloughing-off of tampon material. Needless to say, the treatment was painful and expensive."

"I've had cystitis for years. When I stopped using tampons last year my bladder problems went away. What's the connection?"

We don't really know all the connections. In fact, we don't know much at all about tampons of a "scientific" nature. But we do know, as a result of the blitz of information and speculation about toxic shock syndrome, that tampons are not necessarily safe or innocuous.

Tampons are not sterilized and are produced under unsterile conditions. Food and Drug Administration inspectors have reported finding mineral oil and other contaminants on tampons as they came off the assembly line.

"Deodorant" tampons—actually perfumed tampons—

can cause irritation to the mucosal membrane of the vagina.

Many plastic tampon applicators have sharp cusps that can lacerate vaginal membranes.

Tampon withdrawal strings can act as wicks, carrying bacteria from feces into the vagina, where they may cause infections.

Chemically altered fibers—now used in virtually every tampon on the American market—can be so absorbent that they dry out the vagina, causing it to become irritated and sore.

What all this means is that *tampons have changed*. With the exception of the withdrawal string, all of the above features are relatively new ones—and in one way or another, they affect *nearly every tampon on the market*.

The first deodorant tampon wasn't introduced until 1969.

Plastic tampon inserters were introduced a few years earlier, but they originally had open ends. The "petal" tips with their sharp points, which made their debut in the early seventies, were touted as an "improvement" that facilitated insertion.

In the late thirties and early forties, tampons were sterilized with ethylene oxide gas after they were wrapped. The practice was later abandoned after it was discovered that the gas left a residue on the tampons—yet other, safer methods of sterilization were never substituted.

Possibly the most dramatic change in tampons has been in their fiber content. Tampons were originally made of surgical cotton, rayon (refined from wood), gauze or crepe paper. They gained absorbency by being tightly compressed or crimped. But in the mid-seventies the technology of superabsorbency revolutionized American industry, and makers of menstrual products were quick to catch on to the potential.

"Super slurper" fibers were first used in agriculture to coat seeds and condition soil; they had the unique property of absorbing 300 to 5,000 times their weight in water while holding the water in by forming a gel "pocket." The superabsorbents adapted for tampons (and, by the way, sanitary napkins and diapers) slurped up much less fluid—only 10 to 20 times the fiber weight. But it was their capacity to *retain* fluid that made them so valuable to the tampon industry. Soon chemically altered cotton, rayon and (in the case of Rely tampons) polyester began being substituted for the less-absorbent, unaltered fibers. The question now is: How much absorbency is needed? And how much is too much?

That question hasn't been answered because the tampon companies haven't addressed it. And under current law the federal government cannot set standards for the manufacture of tampons. As a result, questions about tampons are being answered not in the laboratory but at the grocery store checkout counter and in women's homes.

What We Don't Know

Tampons are commonplace in American women's lives. Each month, some 50 million women use them. The tampon industry reaps more than $400 million a year in sales, out of a total "sanitary protection" market of $850 million. It spends some $60 million a year on advertising. Yet for all their ordinariness, for all their acceptance, tampons remain a mystery to the women who use them, to doctors, to the federal government and even to their manufacturers.

Most women who buy and use tampons do so because of advertising, or because of the advice of friends or relatives. They don't know what's in the tampons they buy—because tampon manufacturers aren't required by law to list contents the way cosmetics and over-the-counter drug manufacturers are. As of the date of this writing, only one tampon manufacturer—Playtex, the number-two selling brand in the United States—lists the ingredients of its tampon, and that list doesn't indicate whether the fibers in the tampon are bleached, chemically modified to enhance absorbency, or otherwise altered; and it doesn't give the proportions of the materials in the tampon. The deodorant in Playtex deodorant tampons is listed simply as "fragrance"—a catchall term that may include dozens of substances. The other tampon brands give away even fewer trade secrets, hiding instead behind trademarks such as "Supercotton."

Doctors don't know much about tampons, either. Until recently, the only time a doctor was likely to deal with tampons as a medical problem was when a patient had forgotten to remove one and developed a discharge as a result. Removing a tampon, most doctors agree, is a highly disagreeable chore. "The odor, after a tampon's been forgotten for a couple of weeks, is just awful," one doctor confided. "We have to close off the room." But the routine use of tampons is a subject most doctors rarely bother with. "I send my nurse out to buy them, to have on hand for patients," a male California gynecologist told me. "She buys whatever's on sale." A female Maryland obstetrician recalled that "we were never told anything about tampons in medical school. I learned what I know from advertisements."

The government doesn't know much about tampons, because it's only recently that the government has had any effective means to regulate them. Until 1968, tampons were classified by the Food and Drug Administration as cosmetics—a low-priority category then and now. Since 1968, they've been classed as medical devices, but as "low-priority" ones. Tampons haven't had to meet government standards before going on the market because there were and are no government standards. The FDA can inspect tampon manufacturing facilities, examine books and make recommendations for compliance with the agency's regulations regarding "good manufacturing practices," but it can't require manufacturers to tell the public what they're putting in their tampons. Nor can it require manufacturers to perform any tests for tampon safety before tampons are sold.

Even tampon manufacturers don't know everything there is to know about tampons. Manufacturers seem to rely chiefly on their market surveys in deciding how to design tampons. What their market surveys have been telling them, at least for the last five years, is that women want more absorbent tampons—tampons with less "bypass," as they call leakage in the feminine hygiene business. So tampon companies have been putting more and more absorbent materials in their tampons. But how do the tampon makers measure absorbency? Not with actual menstrual fluid—or even a reasonable facsimile. They test their tampons with saline or gelatin solution—substances that could never be mistaken for menstrual fluid. Consequently, manufacturers don't know how effectively tampons absorb sloughed-off uterine cells, cervical mucus or any of the other components of menstrual "blood."

But because no one else is supplying adequate information about tampons, the woman who chooses to use them has no alternative but to turn to the manufacturers—with all their biases—for tampon facts. Reading advertisements, tampon boxes and package inserts, she acquires all the knowledge she may ever learn about tampons.

Tales From the Tampon Box

All tampons are packaged with some sort of informational material—usage instructions, anatomical diagrams, answers to questions about menstruation, even—recently—warnings about toxic shock syndrome.

What sorts of things is a woman likely to read when she opens a box of tampons?

"Designed by a woman gynecologist."

Tampon companies frequently refer to medical consultants in order to heighten their products' credibility. Notice, however, that those doctors are never named. And if you take the trouble to write or call manufacturers to obtain names of doctors who devised or endorsed their tampons, you'll be politely but firmly told that it's none of your business.

For example, I tried to reach the "woman gynecologist" said to be responsible for the design of o.b. tampons. Personal Products Company, the Johnson and Johnson subsidiary which markets o.b., informed me that she was a "respected European doctor" whose name could not be divulged "because we respect her privacy."

Tampax Incorporated *does* supply the name of the doctor who patented the original Tampax tampon—45 years ago. Since then, though, the fiber content of Tampax tampons has changed so dramatically that it's doubtful their creator would recognize his invention.

Tampon manufacturers' secrecy regarding their medical advisers and researchers isn't limited to the general public. I spoke with a scientist who had been under contract to Kimberly-Clark Corporation—makers of Kotex napkins and tampons—to do a study related to tampon usage. She had tried without success to obtain from Kimberly-Clark the names of other scientists engaged in research in order to discuss her findings with them. Apparently, this scientist told me, this is not the sort of information the corporation wants disseminated—even among the research community.

"Safe for unmarried women."

After all these years, that's still how some tampon manufacturers refer to virgins. Others use similar euphemisms such as "young girls" or "women of all ages." What they're talking about are girls and women whose hymens have not been fully stretched open—something that sometimes (but by no means always) occurs during the first act of sexual intercourse. In fact, some girls and women's hymens have relatively large openings from birth, while others become stretched during strenuous exercise, masturbation or vaginal examination with a speculum.

However, a small yet significant number of virgins do experience difficulty in wearing tampons. In these girls and women, the hymen may divide the vaginal opening roughly in half, or the hymen may have a very small opening. Although they may be able to insert a tampon, once the tampon has expanded inside the vagina it is very painful to remove.

"Can't get lost inside your body."

It's certainly true that the vagina is a "dead end"—it has no opening into the abdomen. Technically, then, a tampon really can't become "lost" inside a woman's body.

Nevertheless, an extraordinary number of women report the experience of a lost tampon. What has usually happened is that the tampon withdrawal string has disappeared inside the vagina—or, occasionally, fallen out—and the tampon itself has lodged high inside one of the vaginal fornices. (See Chapter 2 for a more complete description of female reproductive anatomy.) A woman who is inexperienced with tampons, or who has never explored her vagina through self-examination, may react to this experience as though her body has "swallowed" the tampon. A lot of women in this predicament end up in tears in a doctor's office. "It's a very common thing," a nurse-practitioner in Denver told me. "What's strange is that the women in this situation become so frightened. Rather than relax and try to reach for the tampon, they panic. To them, the vagina is a dark, mysterious place."

Instead of simply telling women that tampons *cannot* become lost inside the vagina, manufacturers could address this sense of doubt and fear in clear, sympathetic terms.

"Safe, fresh scent . . . reduces doubt about intimate odor."

Here's a paradox. All tampons eliminate menstrual odor by preventing menstrual fluid from coming into contact with air and decomposing. Why, then, should fragrance be added to tampons?

Let's let the president of International Playtex, Inc.,

Walter Bregman, explain it. Playtex is currently the only tampon brand on the U.S. market that includes a deodorant version (although Personal Products Company is test-marketing a competitor, Assure! Natural Fit Tampons).

In an October 1980 hearing of the FDA's Ob-Gyn Advisory Panel, Mr. Bregman told his audience that "extensive research revealed to us that this was an element in the tampon which many consumers desire and it is no secret to our competitors that the product today is a highly successful product, because consumers want it and buy it."

In other words: You women were the ones who wanted your vaginas to smell like roses, or bubble gum. Don't blame *us*.

Playtex claims that the fragrance it uses is "proven" safe and nontoxic. Yet the warning on boxes of deodorant Playtex to "discontinue use if sensitivity or irritation occurs" indicates that the manufacturer is aware that there are risks involved in using perfumed tampons. Fragrances are complex substances, and there are documented cases of allergic reactions to them. At least 12 complaints in the FDA's Device Experience Network report burning, itching, rashes and other side effects of perfumed tampons.

In short, deodorant tampons are unnecessary—and they can be dangerous. A growing number of doctors are warning their patients to avoid them, just as they should avoid perfumed douche solutions or "feminine hygiene sprays." A healthy vagina cleans itself, and has a characteristic odor that doesn't need to be covered up with scent. A bad-smelling vaginal discharge is a sign of an infection that needs to be treated—not masked.

Tampon manufacturers provide us with other half-truths and misinformation. The anatomical drawings on package inserts, for example, never include the clitoris or the hymen, and only occasionally the cervix. Drawings of differently shaped hymens would be enormously reassuring to young, virginal girls attempting to insert their first tampon—but you'll never find them in a box of tampons.

What you *will* find is an emphasis on how the menstrual

cycle is a preparation for pregnancy. Certainly that's physiologically accurate. But in women's actual lives, menstruation is experienced much more frequently than pregnancy—if pregnancy is experienced at all—and our menstrual cycles have greater significance to us than for their reproductive potential.

What's In a Tampon?

If you buy eyeliner, its contents will be labeled on the package. If you buy cereal, you know what you're getting—the ingredients are listed on the box. But if you buy tampons, you have no way of knowing what's in them. Federal law does not require tampon manufacturers to list contents, and so far only one company—Playtex—has voluntarily listed ingredients on its tampon boxes.

Since the toxic shock syndrome scare, though, tampon companies have relinquished some of their trade secrets to the federal Centers for Disease Control, and some of that information has dribbled out to the general media. Here's what I've learned about tampon contents, based on published reports, direct observation, and bits of knowledge gleaned from conversations with tampon company spokesmen.

TAMPAX, the number-one selling brand in the United States (and probably the world), accounts for about half of the U.S. tampon market. Tampax manufactures five sizes of tampons: junior, slender, regular, super and super plus. All five versions have cardboard applicators made of spirally wound strips of paper held together with water-soluble glue, and all five have single, waterproofed withdrawal strings stitched down their lengths. Each tampon is individually wrapped in paper. When dunked in water, all Tampax tampons expand longitudinally more than they expand radially. Presumably, they behave in a similar fashion inside a woman's vagina. Perhaps for this reason some women find Tampax tampons too long to be comfortable.

Of the five types of Tampax, according to Tampax medical director Dr. Clayton L. Thomas, only "Super" and the recently revived all cotton "Regular" resembles the original Tampax tampon, patented in the mid-1930s. Super, the bestselling Tampax tampon, is made of a blend of "unmodified cotton and rayon." Original regular, brought back in mid-1981 after having been phased out three years earlier, is made of 100% cotton. Certain substances are added to increase the bonding between the fibers or enhance absorbency; the company does not detail the composition of these substances.

Tampax junior is made entirely of rayon.[1] It is the smallest and least-absorbent Tampax tampon, and although it's available in many stores, Tampax ads rarely refer to it. I was told this is because junior "just isn't absorbent enough for anything but the lightest flows."

Tampax slender regular is made of cotton, rayon and high-absorbency modified carboxymethylcellulose. Like cotton and rayon, carboxymethylcellulose is a type of cellulose. However, it's been chemically treated so that it absorbs many times its own weight in fluid—and holds it in. The modified celluloses used in the agriculture industry can hold as much as 5,000 times their own weight; the carboxymethylcellulose used in tampons is much less absorbent, soaking up only about 10 to 20 times its weight in fluid.

Tampax super plus is made of high-absorbency rayon polyacrylate, a modified form of rayon. It has the same dimensions of Tampax super when dry, but it's capable of absorbing more.

When Tampax slender regular and Tampax super plus are left in glasses of water for about 30 minutes, tiny fibers can be seen drifting away from the tampons and into the water, until the water appears cloudy.

Tampax tampons have been associated with about 5 percent of toxic shock syndrome cases studied by the Centers for Disease Control. Tampax brand tampons have been named in Device Experience Network reports in association with vaginal ulcers, cervical burns and discharge, irritation, spotting, and longer periods of flow.

PLAYTEX tampons account for about 23 percent of the U.S. tampon market. They're made in three sizes—regular, super and super plus—with deodorant versions in each size. All Playtex tampons have polyethylene applicators with six pointed cusps at one end; the deodorant version's applicator is pink, the non-deodorant version's is white. The tampons are individually wrapped in paper.

Playtex tampons are all made of rayon polyacrylate, cotton and "trace" amounts of polysorbate-20, a substance added to synthetic fibers to increase their surface tension, the way—for example—lanolin does in natural wool. The deodorant versions add "fragrance" to the list of ingredients.

The withdrawal string on Playtex tampons is threaded through a hole about half an inch from the end of the tampon. It's easily pulled out—and, in fact, some consumer complaints have addressed this problem. The exterior of a Playtex tampon appears glossy, as though it's coated. When pulled apart, it reveals two overlapping layers of tightly compressed fibers. This design is a selling point in some magazine advertisements that feature a woman customer demanding, "Make mine a double!"

When placed in a glass of water, Playtex tampons swell radially within seconds to fill the entire circumference of the glass. Within half an hour, tiny fibers fill the water.

Playtex tampons were associated by the Centers for Disease Control with about 20 percent of toxic shock syndrome cases studied. Complaints about Playtex in the DEN involve strings that break off or pull out, tampons that fall apart within the vagina, reactions to the fragrance in the deodorant versions, ulcerations and lacerations from the plastic inserter.

KOTEX tampons make up about 10 percent of the market. They're made in two versions: stick and "security" (formerly "heavy-duty"). Both versions come in two sizes, regular and super.

The stick in the stick tampons is made of wound paper. It's pushed into a depression in the tampon much as a lollipop stick would be. The tampons are individually wrapped in cellophane. The withdrawal string is threaded and looped through a hole about half an inch from the end of the tampon and knotted on its end. Both regular and super sizes are made of cotton, rayon and superabsorbent modified carboxymethylcellulose. They're very highly compressed and, when dry, very hard—it's virtually impossible to pull one apart. They expand radially and longitudinally in water into an oblong shape, and after several minutes begin shedding short fibers.

Kotex security tampons come in applicators made of polyethylene and polypropylene plastic, and they're wrapped in paper. There are five cusps on the end of the applicator. The tampons themselves are made of the same materials as the stick tampons, but they're less compressed and pull apart readily to reveal an "overwrap" that covers fiber and small chips—possibly the carboxymethylcellulose. The withdrawal string is attached in the same way as in the stick tampons. Security tampons expand in water into an oblong shape and begin shedding fibers soon after immersion.

Kotex tampons were associated with about 2 percent of toxic shock syndrome cases. Complaints in the DEN regarding Kotex involve mostly lacerations—both from the plastic applicator and from the stick applicator.

O.B. tampons represent about 9 percent of the U.S. market. They have no applicator. Each tampon is individually wrapped in cellophane, and the tampon is inserted with a finger.

o.b.'s makers, Personal Products Company, claim that no modified superabsorbent materials are used in their product. Instead, the rolled construction of the cotton and rayon layers supposedly enhances absorbency simply through its design. o.b. comes in three sizes—regular, super and super plus. Each size, when inserted into a glass of water, swells into a "barrel" shape within seconds, and sheds long fibers into the water. The blue withdrawal string is knotted at one end and draped over the tampon material so that it's enclosed when the tampon is rolled during manufacture.

o.b. tampons were associated with 2 percent of toxic shock syndrome cases. Consumers have complained in the DEN that the tampon material falls apart inside the vagina, and at least one doctor has had to assist "several virginal adolescents" in whom o.b. tampons had become trapped behind the hymen.

ASSURE! NATURAL FIT TAMPONS are currently being test-marketed by Personal Products. Marketing slogans promise "a whole new attitude toward your period." Assure comes in regular, super and super plus sizes, with a very sweet-smelling deodorant version in each size. The tampon is contained in a plastic applicator with four rounded cusps on its end; the entire tampon is encased in a plastic wrapper. The materials of the tampon are still a secret, but the construction closely resembles o.b.'s "rolled" design. The withdrawal string is attached in the same way as o.b.'s. Women in Rochester, New York, a test market, have filed a number of complaints claiming that Assure fell apart inside their vaginas.

PURSETTES, which has the smallest share of the tampon market—just 1 percent—has been around for nearly 30 years with few substantial changes. Like o.b., it has no applicator and is individually wrapped in cellophane. It consists of a nonwoven rayon overwrap that covers a layer of rayon fibers; the whole tampon is folded once across its width. The tip of each Pursettes tampon is coated with a water-soluble food-grade polyethylene oxide that becomes sticky when moistened. The waxed cotton withdrawal string is looped through a hole in the tampon near one end. In water, Pursettes expands through its width, and sheds in both strands and small chunks of fiber. It tends to drip considerably more than other tampons. It comes in two absorbency sizes, regular and plus.

To date, there has been one reported case of toxic shock syndrome in a Pursettes user. No complaints in the Device Experience Network are connected with Pursettes.

RELY tampons were officially withdrawn from the market by their maker, Procter & Gamble, in September 1980. However, their recall has not been monitored by the FDA, and supplies may still be available in some stores. In addition, there have been unconfirmed reports that Rely is still being sold outside of the United States. Procter & Gamble is offering a full refund for the return of any remaining Rely tampons.

For the record, Rely represented a revolutionary change in tampon design. Instead of being made of compressed fibers, it consisted of a nonwoven polyester bag loosely filled with tiny polyester sponges and chips of carboxymethylcellulose. The applicator was made of plastic with four sharp cusps on one end, and the tampons were individually wrapped in paper. The withdrawal string was knotted around the end of the bag. The tampon was very soft to the touch, and when dunked in water it expanded dramatically through its radius. It retained liquid to a remarkable degree—according to ads, as much as 17 times its weight.

Rely was withdrawn from sale after it was associated with 71 percent of toxic shock syndrome cases studied by the Centers for Disease Control. Other consumer complaints about Rely, documented in the DEN, concerned lacerations from the inserter, difficulty in removing, and disintegration of the tampon inside the vagina.

Aside from the known components of tampons, other substances have been considered by tampon manufacturers—and possibly put to use. Women Health International, a Washington, D.C.–based research group, found patent applications filed by various tampon manufacturers for the use of talc and polyvinyl alcohol (among other substances) in inserters and tampons.[2] Talc has been associated with cancer of the cervix,[3] and polyvinyl alcohol sponges have produced inflammations and lacerations when inserted into the vaginas of laboratory animals.[4] What these materials might do—or have done—when inserted into the vaginas of human females is still a matter for serious speculation.

NOTES

1. This and other information about tampon contents is adapted from "What's in the Tampons That Are Still on the Market?" *Medical World News* 21:9, November 10, 1980.

2. Charlotte Oram and Judith Beck, "Forty-Seven Years Later—Are Tampons Really Safe?", p. 8.

3. W.J. Henderson et. al., "Talc and Carcinoma of the Ovary and Cervix," *The Journal of Obstetrics and Gynaecology of the British Commonwealth*, 78:, p. 266 March 1971.

4. M. Chaupal et al., "Reaction of Vaginal Tissue of Rabbits to Inserted Sponges Made of Various Materials," *Journal of Biomedical Materials Research* 13:1, January 1979.

CHAPTER 2

A Woman's Body

The Basic Parts

A detailed discussion of human female anatomy is beyond the scope—and the point—of this book. But in order to fully understand how tampons work, it's important to understand the function of a few anatomical features: the vagina, the cervix, the hymen and the perineal (between anus and urinary opening) area.

The *vagina* is frequently described as a potential space rather than an actual space, not only because its size and shape vary so much from woman to woman, but also because each woman's vagina is capable, on the right occasion, of enlarging to accommodate a tampon, a penis, or the body of a baby during delivery. The vagina is also capable of contracting vigorously, as during orgasm. There is no relationship between the size of a woman's vagina and her overall body size, but a woman who has borne many children may have a vagina with less elasticity than a woman who has never given birth.

"The great silent area of the pelvis," one poetically in-

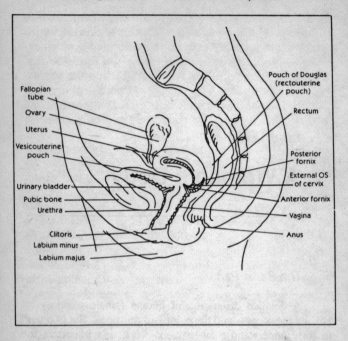

Fallopian tube
Ovary
Uterus
Vesicouterine pouch
Urinary bladder
Pubic bone
Urethra
Clitoris
Labium minus
Labium majus

Pouch of Douglas (rectouterine pouch)
Rectum
Posterior fornix
External OS of cervix
Anterior fornix
Vagina
Anus

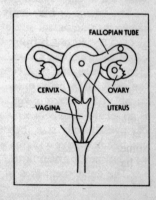

FALLOPIAN TUBE
CERVIX
VAGINA
OVARY
UTERUS

Anatomical drawings in tampon package inserts, like this one from o.b. tampons, usually omit important features such as the hymen and clitoris. Compare it with the above drawing from Biology of Women.

clined doctor called the vagina, and there's some truth to his metaphor. Almost all of the nerve endings in the vagina are concentrated near the opening (or *introitus*), which explains why a correctly inserted tampon can hardly be felt. A tampon can't ever really be "lost" inside the vagina, because it has no opening into the abdominal cavity, and the cervical opening (os), which extends down into the vagina, can't be pushed open except by medical instruments or, again, by a baby during delivery.

The area of the vagina around the *cervix* (the cervix is the lower part of the uterus which extends down into the vagina) forms four projections of unequal size and shape, called the anterior, right and left lateral and posterior fornices. ("Fornix" is Latin for "horn," which is roughly what they look like.) During a manual pelvic examination, it's these fornices that are probed in order to feel the positions of the uterus, ovaries and Fallopian tubes. Occasionally a tampon may get pushed deep into one of the fornices, especially if a second one has been inserted. It's still possible to retrieve it, but some women find that a doctor's or nurse's aid has to be enlisted.

The best way to understand the relationship of the cervix to the vagina is through self-examination, a technique made accessible by the women's self-care movement. Using an inexpensive plastic speculum—a device that holds apart the vaginal walls—a mirror and a strong source of light, a woman can see her own cervix and vaginal walls, and take note of changes or abnormalities. Self examination is taught at women's health clinics. If one doesn't exist in your area, you can start by asking your doctor to let you hold a mirror during an office exam.

The *hymen* is nature's mystery—and perhaps more than menstruation itself, woman's true "curse." It has no anatomical or physiological function except to be destroyed, yet in nearly every culture in the world it's regarded with something approaching awe. In some places it can be said to have an economic function, for in its absence a bride's "market value" plummets to nil. A thin membrane that surrounds the vaginal opening but almost never blocks it completely, the hymen is widely believed to be a symbol of virginity. In fact, some girls and women have hymens that are sufficiently stretched (from tampon use, habitual douching or masturbation), ruptured (from horseback riding or other strenuous activity) or wide enough since birth to allow them to experience their first intercourse without painful "defloration" or bleeding. Other young women have their hymens painlessly widened by their physicians in order to prevent needless trauma in the future. Fragments of hymen remain after intercourse and even after childbirth.

Almost all hymens have openings to allow menstrual blood to pass through, and in nearly every case, those openings are large enough for tampons to be inserted and removed as well. Exceptions include virgins whose hymens have a septum that divides the introitus to the vagina in half. One family practitioner told me that in the last two years she'd seen two patients, both young teenage girls, with this irregularity; in both cases, the girls had inserted tampons that had expanded inside their vaginas and then they had found them nearly impossible to remove—the tampons had become wedged against the hymen. With doctors becoming better informed about tampon use among "unmarried girls" (as the tampon company brochures still like to call virgins), it's to be hoped that they'll give their young patients clearer advice before emergencies develop.

The *perineum* doesn't seem, at first, to have much to do with the reproductive organs. Yet it plays a crucial role in the "sanitaryness" of "sanitary protection." Early champions of tampons pointed out that sanitary napkins, which bridge the entire perineal area, were breeding grounds for bacteria carried in feces. In addition, glands in the perineal area secrete perspiration and sebaceous (waxy) substances that can contribute to the development of diseases like cystitis (chronic and extremely painful bladder inflammation), vaginitis and yeast infections, especially in warm, humid climates where the organisms that cause these diseases thrive anyway.

But napkins aren't the only culprit. The string on commercial tampons also hangs down into the perineal region, and it, too, can pick up bacteria from waste products. It may even be a more efficient disease carrier than a napkin, because it is capable of "wicking" bacteria up into the vagina. Tampon users who suffer from chronic bouts with vaginal or urinary infections might try cutting the string short—or discontinuing tampons altogether—to see whether the string has been a factor in their illness.

The Menstrual Cycle

All healthy women—in fact, all healthy female primates—menstruate between the ages of puberty and menopause—unless, of course, they happen to be pregnant. (It may take more than a month for menstruation to resume after childbirth, but, contrary to a commonly held belief, breastfeeding does not indefinitely postpone the return of ovulation—or of menstrual periods.)

Aside from that generalization, however, there is very little one can say about the menstrual cycle that applies to *all* women of menstruating age. For example, the "normal" length of a menstrual cycle—the time span from the first day of bleeding in one period to the first day of bleeding in the next—is often said to be 28 days. But that figure is simply a statistical average, and it's probably caused more anxiety and doubt among women than any other piece of information about their bodies. In fact, it's safe to say that no woman in the world has ever had "perfect" 28-day cycles throughout her fertile life.

Likewise, the "average" woman menstruates for approximately five days during each cycle—but she is just as likely to flow for two, or three, or eight (and just as "normal" if she does). Illness, emotional distress, fatigue, travel or malnutrition may trigger—or postpone—menstruation, depending on the individual. I know a post-menopausal woman who claims that air travel used to cause her to menstruate earlier than she'd expected, but flight attendants who regularly crisscross the country or the globe may stop menstruating altogether for periods of time, as may some women who work at night or in photographic darkrooms.

Menstrual bleeding (or *menses*) is both the end of one menstrual cycle and the beginning of another. Although the first day of bleeding is considered Day One of a given menstrual cycle, it represents the completion of a complex chain of hormonal events that was designed to lead to conception—but didn't.

In order for normal menstruation to occur, *ovulation* must first have taken place. (The exceptions usually happen during early puberty, when menstrual periods are just beginning, and around the menopause, when they're stopping). Ovulation is the release of an egg from the follicle, or bundle of cells, that has surrounded it inside one or the other ovary. In some women, the ovaries take turns releasing eggs; in others, there's no regular pattern. Some women experience ovulation as a cramp on the left or right side of the abdomen or lower back. The medical term for this is a German word, *mittelschmerz*, which means "middle pain" ("middle" refers to the middle of the cycle, not the middle of the body). Sometimes there's an accompanying discharge, which may have a little blood in it. This phenomenon is called by a hybrid word, "mittelstaining."

As the follicle matures in the ovary in the first half of the cycle, it produces estrogen, a hormone, that signals the uterine lining (endometrium) to grow, thicken, and create glands. After the egg is released and begins traveling through the fallopian tube (oviduct), the follicle it left behind, now called the corpus luteum, switches from producing only estrogen to producing a second hormone as well, progesterone. Progesterone causes the glands in the uterine lining to start secreting nourishment for the egg, which may or may not become fertilized during its tubal trip. Progesterone also brings about an increase in the blood supply to the uterus, so that the endometrium becomes lush and velvety.

When fertilization fails to occur, the corpus luteum stops secreting hormones. This abrupt drop in hormone production is thought to account for the mood shift many women experience several days before menstruation, and it may also explain why some women have skin problems (from pimples to herpes) and are more prone to infections and colds just before they menstruate.

With no hormones telling it to continue preparations for pregnancy, the uterine "nest" stops growing. Instead, it begins to disintegrate. Over the next three to seven days, (more or less), all but about a third of this lining oozes out through the cervical opening, through the vaginal canal and out of the body. The remnant of the lining left behind becomes the basis for the next cycle's lining.

Menstrual fluid is commonly thought of as "blood," but in fact it's a lot more—and a lot different. Besides blood, which makes up something over half its content, menstrual fluid also contains the glandular secretions of the endometrium and sloughed-off cells from the uterine lining itself. Unlike blood from any other part of the body, menstrual blood does not clot unless the flow is very heavy. What may appear to be a clot in a normal flow is actually a plug of red blood cells, mucus and glandular secretions, including proteins. Menstrual blood has no odor until it makes contact with bacteria in the air (and, when "sanitary" pads are used, with bacteria from around the anus and urinary opening). This is why tampons eliminate odor—and why "deodorant" in tampons is an unnecessary addition.

Exactly how much lining is shed each cycle—the amount of flow—is subject to some dispute, mainly because it's not the easiest thing to measure. If you've ever tried a menstrual "cup," (Tassette or Tassaway) with its standard capacity of one ounce, you've probably been surprised at how small the volume of flow actually is, compared with what it may seem to be. According to estimates in the medical literature, the normal range of flow is about 20 milliliters (about a tablespoon) to about 150 milliliters (about seven and a half tablespoons, or 3 ounces) for the entire menstrual period, with as much as half the total flow occurring on the first day. Flows of greater than 150 milliliters are sometimes called *menorrhagia*.

Even seven tablespoons is not a great deal of blood loss and the majority of women are able to part with it without suffering anemia. But even a flow of only three tablespoons can seem like a lot of blood because it is not lost gradually but rather stops and starts throughout menses. That's one reason for "leaks" while tampons are worn; anatomical variations in the shape of the vagina are another.

Most medical researchers agree that menstrual blood is sterile—free of disease-causing organisms. But one scientist proposed in 1973 that menstrual blood could carry certain blood-borne diseases—specifically, viral hepatitis, mononucleosis and syphilis—while leaving the carrier (the menstruating woman) free of symptoms. Writing in the "Hypothesis" column of *The Lancet*, the prestigious British medical journal, Scott Mazzur of the Institute for Cancer Research in Philadelphia suggested that taboos regarding menstruating women (in some cultures, they are virtually isolated and forbidden to prepare food, have sexual contact or care for children) may be "a subconscious adaptation to disease."[1] It's interesting to reflect that connections between menstrual blood and venereal disease are rife in folklore. However, Mazzur's theory has never been tested, and it remains an intriguing—and disturbing—conjecture.

"Those In-Between Days"

A visitor from another galaxy who read current American advertising for tampons, sanitary napkins and mini-pads would probably come away imagining that the overriding characteristic of womanhood was leakiness. This tampon gives you "snug fit against leaks"; that pantiliner "can make you feel better 25 days a month" because it absorbs "*between*-period discharge." Just what is all this wetness, and where is it coming from?

Some vaginal discharge is perfectly normal throughout the nonbleeding days of the menstrual cycle—it's the vagina's way of cleansing itself. Estrogen manufactured by the ovaries causes the cells of the vaginal epithelium, or lining, to proliferate rapidly. As they grow, these cells accumulate glycogen (a form of glucose, which is a sugar), which is in turn broken down by bacteria called Doderlein's bacilli, which are part of the normal bacterial inhabitants of the vagina. The normal vaginal discharge consists of Doderlein's bacilli (lactobacilli), sloughed-off cells from the vaginal lining, and a little cervical mucus produced by the cervical glands. The action of the Doderlein's bacilli changes the vaginal glycogen into lactic acid, and this acidity is responsible for protecting the vagina from alien bacteria and the infections they can cause.

Some women notice a marked change in the quality of their cervical mucus right around the time of ovulation— midway between periods. The mucus becomes stretchy, transparent and smooth, rather like egg white, all of which permits sperm to travel unhindered through the vagina and into the uterus. Sometimes this cervical mucus is prolific enough to be experienced as a slight, clear discharge—once again, a perfectly normal phenomenon that some women learn to welcome because it helps them identify their fertile period. In fact, "natural" birth control—sometimes called the Billings or symptothermal method—relies on observations of cervical mucus and other body signals to let a woman know when she's likely to conceive.

Other *vaginal* discharges are caused by intrauterine devices (IUDs) or by changes in hormonal levels, caused either by medications (including antibiotics or birth control pills) or by infection or illness. Some IUD wearers experience breakthrough bleeding, or spotting, when they're not menstruating. What this means in the long run is still being disputed, but certainly any heavy intermenstrual bleeding should be immediately checked out with a physician. Other IUD wearers notice a somewhat heavier "normal" discharge throughout their cycles. It's speculated that this may be caused by the IUD's irritation of the uterine lining, setting up a constant, low-level infection.

Antibiotics, which kill helpful bacteria along with harmful ones, may promote yeast and other discharge-producing infections in the vagina.

If you must take certain medicines or the Pill, some discharge will probably be part of your life. Cotton underwear may be sufficiently absorbent to keep you comfortable. Avoid nylon underwear though, and choose pantyhose with a cotton crotch: nylon traps heat and moisture which encourage bacteria to grow.

Infectious discharges are another story: They're a sign of an imbalance between helpful and harmful organisms in the body. To cause a vaginal discharge, they may originate in the vagina, in the cervix, in the uterus or in the Fallopian tubes.

Vaginal infections (collectively called vaginitis) include Trichomoniasis, candida albicans (also known as yeast or monilia) and nonspecific vaginitis. "Trich" produces a thin, foamy, foul-smelling, yellowish-green or gray discharge; it's a sexually transmitted infection caused by a parasite that prefers alkaline environments such as the vagina around menstruation (blood is slightly alkaline). Vinegar douches can keep the discharge under control, but usually prescription drugs are needed. Tampons should *not* be used while the infection is being treated.

Yeast infections create thick, white, "cheesy" discharges that itch and burn; they're more widespread than Trich because the fungus that causes them needs only mildly acidic surroundings to grow to unhealthy numbers. Treatment is usually a vaginal cream or suppository, which can itself be pretty "leaky."

Nonspecific vaginitis may produce a white or yellow discharge, along with frequent and painful urination, lower back pain and cramps. Sulfa creams and suppositories are generally prescribed, although antibiotics by mouth are sometimes the preferred treatment. Like "Trich," nonspecific vaginitis is sexually transmitted.

Some gynecologists feel that the use of tampons during a bout of vaginitis is a bad idea because the tampon dams up an infectious discharge that the body is trying to rid itself of. In addition, some doctors speculate that tampons may somehow change the pH (acidity or alkalinity) of the vagina. Yet other doctors have claimed that tampons *relieve* the symptoms of vaginitis by preventing the discharge from making contact with, and thus irritating, the vulva and outer vaginal lips.[2] And one doctor has even published his opinion, based on "repeated observations in the human female," that tampons *cause* vaginitis through a combination of foreign-body reaction to the tampon material and introduction of harmful organisms during insertion.[3] Most doctors probably just don't know, and it probably doesn't occur to most patients to ask. Certainly using tampons to hide the discharge is not a very good idea, since the nature of the discharge itself is a clue to the nature of the infection. And recent medical reports show that women who wear tampons continuously to absorb discharge, seem to be prone to ulcerations (sores) in their vaginas (see Chapter 3).

A *cervical* discharge (which eventually flows out of the vaginal opening) may be caused by cervical erosion. This is a sore on the cervix near the cervical os (opening); it's usually painless (and very common), but it can produce a white, unpleasant-smelling discharge. If the discharge is sufficiently thick, it can cause temporary infertility. If you or your doctor or nurse detects an erosion during a pelvic examination, a Pap smear should be ordered to see whether it's cancerous. If it proves not to be, some doctors will advise that you leave it alone, while others will prescribe a sulfa cream. Cautery with silver nitrate or cryosurgery may be used for severe cases during the course of treatment. The possible connection between tampons and cervical erosion was investigated in several studies during the thirties and forties, when tampons were new on the market, and no relationship was found. However, there have been no new studies since synthetic materials began being widely used in tampons.

Gonorrhea may also cause a cervical discharge, greenish in color, which can spread from the vagina to the anus. Because this discharge is easily mistaken for discharges from less serious vaginal infections, it's important to get a gonorrhea culture when seeing a health professional for *any* genital irritation.

Discharges are also associated with *uterine* infections, including endometritis and pelvic inflammatory disease (PID). Endometritis is an inflammation of the uterine lining, and is thought to be sometimes caused by an IUD; it may create a thick, bad-smelling cervical discharge. The treatment includes antibiotics and frequently removal of the IUD.

PID (Pelvic Inflammatory Disease) is a serious illness that may involve the uterus, Fallopian tubes or ovaries, or all three. It has been associated with IUD use as well as with gonorrhea and other bacterial infection. It usually causes pelvic pain, often very intense, and may lead to sterility. Fever frequently is present also. Irregular non-menstrual bleeding—including spotting and passing clots—and a foul discharge are associated with PID. Treatment may include antibiotics, bed rest and abstinence from sexual intercourse; in some cases, surgery is required.

After an abortion or the delivery of a child, a woman will have a different sort of discharge. For several days after a safe and successful abortion, a woman will have a bloody discharge that resembles a menstrual period. Excessively heavy bleeding may be a sign that the uterus has been perforated or that not all of its contents have been removed. Notify your doctor or a hospital at once if this occurs. To prevent post-abortion infections, *don't use tampons* for the first 10 days; douches and intercourse should also be avoided for this period.

Post-delivery discharge is called *lochia*, and lasts for several weeks. A study published in 1962 [4] found that after the tenth day postpartum, when the cervix was observed to be closed again, it was safe for new mothers to wear tampons. The authors felt that tampons had the advantage over sanitary napkins because they did not press on the tender area where episiotomy (incision between vagina and anus to facilitate delivery) had been performed. However, the second edition of *Our Bodies, Ourselves,* [5] published in 1976, advises that new mothers wait "several weeks" before using tampons. If the cervix is still open when a tampon is inserted, there's a chance that bacteria or even tampon fibers could be introduced into the uterus, causing serious infection.

At what other times do women wear tampons? The answers are varied and sometimes surprising. Some women say they like to wear tampons when they don't wear underwear. One woman said she wore tampons for what she called "P.I.D." *Not* pelvic inflammatory disease, she hastened to add—"post-intercourse drip." She has our sympathies, but she might want to know that although semen has very little odor when it's fresh, it can acquire a very pungent smell after it's been dammed up by a tampon for several hours.

Another woman told me that she and her friends used to insert tampons several hours before intercourse—"so they'd be lubricated"—and leave them in to provide a "tighter fit" for their partners. "This was back in the early seventies—amazing what we used to do before we woke up!" Needless to say, a tampon left in the vagina during intercourse can create a very abrasive experience for both partners.

In fact, the best advice is to avoid using tampons except during menstruation—which was what they were created for. As we'll see, the longer tampons are worn during times other than active menstruation, the greater the risk of medical problems.

NOTES

1. Scott Mazzur, "Menstrual Blood as a Vehicle of Australia-Antigen Transmission," *The Lancet* 7806:749, April 7, 1973.

2. Robert N. Rutherford, A. Lawrence Banks, and Wallace A. Coburn, "Tampons in Relief of Symptomatic Vaginitis," *Pacific Medicine and Surgery* 74:314, November–December 1966.

3. Daniel L. Maguire, Jr., "Tampon Vaginitis," *The Journal of the South Carolina Medical Association,* 62:432, November 1966.

4. R.N. Rutherford, A. Lawrence Banks and W.A. Coburn, "Intravaginal Tampons for the Postpartum Patient," *Obstetrics and Gynecology*, 19:781 June 1962.

5. Boston Women's Health Book Collective, *Our Bodies, Ourselves*, second edition, New York, Simon and Schuster, 1976.

CHAPTER 3

"Invented by a Doctor": A Medical and Social History of Tampons

"New Menstruation Toilet"

For most of us, it's difficult to remember or imagine life before tampons. We tend to forget that it's been less than 50 years since the first disposable tampon with an applicator was marketed. Yet we need to keep in mind just how revolutionary that development was.

In 1936, when Tampax Incorporated introduced its "civilized solution to the problem of sanitary protection," even disposable sanitary napkins were still considered an innovation: They'd been on the American market for less than 20 years. A large number of women were still using clean rags to absorb their menstrual flow, boiling them after each period. Menstruation and menstrual products were not discussed in the popular media; sanitary napkin and belt advertisements in women's magazines (the only periodicals that accepted them) were discreet to the point of mystery and confined to the back pages, along with the school and camp directories.

Yet although the overwhelming majority of women used

external napkins of some sort—Kotex was already becoming a generic name—some women did use tampons. They made them at home out of surgical cotton, cutting strips to size and rolling them tightly for insertion, or they bought natural sea sponges at cosmetics or art supply stores and trimmed them into reusable tampons. But these women belonged to an exclusive margin of society; they tended to be actresses, models, athletes or prostitutes—all dubious professions, in the eyes of "respectable" women. Remember, too, that well into the twentieth century some girls and women who were caught masturbating had their clitorises or ovaries surgically removed as a "cure." It's easy to see how, given such attitudes, tampons might be viewed as immoral.

They hadn't always been. In fact, although the written history of menstrual products is even more scanty than the literature on menstruation itself, there is evidence of tampon use throughout history in a multitude of cultures. The oldest printed medical document, papyrus ebers, refers to the use of soft papyrus tampons by Egyptian women in the fifteenth century B.C. Roman women used wool tampons. Women in ancient Japan fashioned tampons out of paper, held them in place with a bandage, and changed them 10 to 12 times a day. Traditional Hawaiian women used the furry part of a native fern called hapu'u; and grasses, mosses and other plants are still used by women in parts of Asia and Africa.

In the United States, though, it took a male doctor to come up with a satisfactory "solution" to the "problem." It seemed that there were ever-increasing numbers of women who were "respectable" yet active, too, and to them the sanitary napkin-and-belt appurtenance was a burden. Horseback riding, bicycling and, of course, swimming were awkward if not completely proscribed, and jobs that demanded physical exertion were often out of the question.

One woman in such a situation was Myrtle Haas, a Denver nurse who found sanitary napkins uncomfortably chafing while she was on duty. Her husband, Dr. Earle Haas, resolved to do something to help her. Adapting the device used after surgery to absorb bleeding in body orifices (nose, vagina, anus), he created a menstrual tampon out of compressed surgical cotton. Down its length was stitched a heavy, waterproofed cord; the whole thing was contained in a two-part applicator made out of spiral strips of cardboard bound together with nontoxic glue.

Dr. Haas obtained a patent for his device in 1933, and not long afterward, drug and department stores began selling it. In 1936, a brand-new company, Tampax Incorporated, bought the Haas patent and launched a massive advertising campaign.

Within a year, the Tampax tampon was a success, and imitations flourished. In June 1937, Tampax could boast in a *Good Housekeeping* ad that "hundreds of letters of praise and gratitude" had poured in to the company. "In the last year thousands and thousands of women have been using Tampax regularly," the ad went on. "Their letters tell us daily of the new freedom, the new comfort, the new daintiness, Tampax has made possible." If women still harbored doubts, both the advertisement and the package itself informed them that the product was "accepted for advertising by the Journal of the American Medical Association." Only the box was pictured in the ad (along with the price, 35 cents for a box of 10); by the war years unwrapped tampons would be depicted as well.

The fact that "thousands and thousands of women" were switching to "internal protection" did not escape public notice. Clergymen rushed to denounce tampons as agents of defloration and general wickedness, the idea being that if a young woman got used to inserting tampons into her vagina, she'd sooner or later conceive the idea of inserting even more pernicious devices. Doctors' reactions ranged from skeptical to disapproving—the author of one gynecological textbook called tampons a "menace."

For better or for worse, though, tampons were taken seriously, as they could continue to be through World War II. The problem was that no one had taken them very seriously *before* they were placed on the marketplace. In fact, the first discussions of tampons in American medical literature did not appear until March 1938—some five years after commercial tampons began to be sold.

That study, "Vaginal Tamponage for Catamenial [menstrual] Protection,"[1] was written by Lloyd Arnold, M.D., and Marie Hagele, a nurse, and was funded by the International Cellucotton Products Corporation, which at the time manufactured Kotex sanitary napkins and Fibs(!) tampons. The aim of the research was to "determine the efficiency of tampons in collecting the catamenial discharge of normal women." Ninety-five women and three makes of tampons (none of them named) were studied; the women wore both tampons and sanitary pads, which the researchers weighed to see how much fluid the tampon collected, and how much leaked onto the napkin.

The results were hardly encouraging to the fledgling tampon industry. Nine out of ten women needed a pad in addition to a tampon for most of the duration of their periods. In addition, urine was found on a large number of tampons (presumably because they weren't inserted high enough into the vagina), and 18 women said they experienced a "gush" of blood immediately after removing a tampon.

Arnold and Hagele's conclusions were understandably cautious. "Tampons are foreign bodies in the vagina," they wrote. "We do not know from experience how susceptible the vaginal mucosa [mucous membrane] may be to repeated irritation. When tampons are used regularly during the menstrual period, periodic examination of the vagina should be made to ascertain whether the mucosa remains normal."

Apparently their advice was heeded, for over the next decade no fewer than 11 reports on tampons were published in medical journals. It was a concentration of interest that would not be duplicated or even approached until the news of toxic shock syndrome once more gave doctors reason to consider the tampon.

In the thirties and early forties, medical opinion was divided on tampons, with "forward-thinking" physicians recommending them wholeheartedly while more conservative doctors waxed eloquent in condemning them. The controversy raged in the letters column of the *British Medical Journal* for three months (November 1938–January 1939).[2] A Dr. E. Lawton Moss of London opened the discussion gruffly, under the headline "New Menstruation Toilet." "During the last few years," wrote Dr. Moss, "I have often been asked by young women whether I considered this new practice of plugging the vagina with absorbent tampons instead of using sanitary pads advisable and healthy. My reply is that it is not at all a good thing to do, because vaginal plugs become very offensive and infected even when introduced by the surgeon under the best aseptic technique, and when introduced by a woman herself . . . the dammed-up blood in the vagina forms a perfect culture medium, and a profuse growth of septic organisms results." The consequences, he added, were "likely" to include vaginitis, cervicitis and bacterial infections, "with quite a possibility of sterility following." He concluded with a plea: "I think it is only fair to the female public to give some advice on the subject, or is it a matter for the Ministry of Health?"

There's no record of the Ministry of Health taking up the banner, but other British doctors did respond to Dr. Moss's battle cry. A Leicester physician offered supporting testimony of a "particularly bad vaginal and cervical infection which the patient herself attributed [to tampons]." But other doctors thought the tampon concept was basically sound. A woman doctor from London, after dismissing sponge tampons as "repellent" (because they were reusable) and commercial cotton tampons as uncomfortable (albeit "sanitary"), endorsed the do-it-yourself tampon made at home out of cotton wool. An Exeter doctor also approved of that method, claiming to have recommended the "self-made plug" for "upwards of fourteen years to a wide range of patients and friends, and I have never encountered any untoward results."

Apparently some British women still follow this practice. But on this side of the Atlantic, the temptation to buy a ready-made product eventually overcame the desire for an individual (and more economical) solution. Tampon brands proliferated and competed in the pages of women's magazines. By 1942, according to a study in *Consumers Reports* (later called *Consumer Reports*), there were nine major brands on the market. Most were made of crimped or compressed cotton, although a few used crepe paper as well.[3]

The trend among doctors—at least those doctors who contributed to medical journals—was to view tampons as harmless, and to reassure women that they could use them confidently. It should come as no surprise that those doctors who undertook clinical studies were often funded by tampon manufacturers.

For example, a study funded by Tampax Incorporated and published in 1942 looked at only 25 women.[4] All of them were given Tampax tampons, which by this time were manufactured in three sizes—junior, regular and super. At the end of the four-month study, the researchers found "not a single instance" of "any evidence of local irritation brought about by the use of the tampons." There was also no bladder irritation, no "appreciable" increase in bacteria in the vagina and cervix, and no difference in vaginal and cervical pH. "The evidence is conclusive," the authors wrote, "that the tampon method of menstrual hygiene is safe, comfortable and not prejudicial to health."

These findings were, however, in direct contradiction to a report published three years earlier in a Swedish medical journal. Two physicians had found three cases of colpitis (vaginitis) which they attributed to the use of Tampax tampons, and they concluded that tampons were unhygienic.[5]

And there were questions raised about tampons even in otherwise favorable reports. A woman health professional wrote in the *British Medical Journal* in 1942 that although tampons eliminated menstrual odor and permitted "complete freedom of movement," they were capable of causing local irritation of the cervix or vagina. Besides, she wrote, "it is difficult for virgins to use an internal pad without causing partial or total rupture of the hymen with regular use. The importance of rupture has only forensic significance, but it is worth considering from the individual standpoint."[6]

The virginity issue, so quaint today, was a serious and significant one all the way through the 1950s. On the one hand, the American entry into World War II gave women more weight in the economy than they had ever before enjoyed, as they entered jobs and roles (such as breadwinner) that had previously been occupied mostly by men. Ads for menstrual products during the war adopted a no-nonsense tone that stressed practical issues such as efficiency and comfort. On the other hand, old moral standards did not automatically wither away, and both men and women were still preoccupied with the "forensic"—in other words, economic—value of the intact hymen.

The 1942 *Consumers Reports* study neatly embodies this conflict. Consumers Union tested 37 sanitary pads and nine tampons for "all-round utility"; women were surveyed to determine how many times they changed pads or tampons (at least four or five times a day, it turned out), and the tampons themselves were tested both for speed of absorption and for total absorption. The technical aspects of the report are matter-of-fact and highly informative; we learn, for example, that under wartime price controls a box of a dozen tampons (the most commonly found package size) cost as little as 20 cents and as much as 45 cents (for Wix brand tampons). Yet moralistic attitudes crept in. Although the article acknowledged that "no thorough clinical study of the safety of tampons has yet been reported," it passed along the unproven hypothesis that tampons dam up the menstrual flow, possibly causing uterine and tubal infections. And the old virginity taboo persisted, discreetly veiled: "Since insertion of tampons is necessary," the report primly advised, "most gynecologists recommend their use only by married women."

But doctors could be invoked to sell tampons as well as to warn their patients away from them. Meds tampons, manufactured by the makers of Modess sanitary napkins,

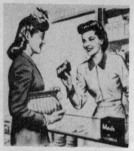

"for real COMFORT, try Meds internal protection!"

Now you can enjoy all the freedom and convenience of this modern method PLUS the special Meds features perfected by a woman doctor.

- Meds are made of real COTTON—soft and super-absorbent for extra comfort.
- Meds alone have the "SAFETY-WELL"—designed for your extra protection.
- Meds' easy-to-use APPLICATORS are dainty, efficient, and disposable.

Meds
only 20¢

FOR 10 IN APPLICATORS

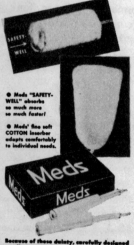

- Meds "SAFETY-WELL" absorbs so much more so much faster!
- Meds' fine soft COTTON inserber adapts comfortably to individual needs.

Because of these dainty, carefully designed applicators, Meds inserbers are easy-to-use!

During World War II, tampon ads like this one for Meds (which appeared in Good Housekeeping in June 1945) stressed practical features such as absorbency. Pictures of unwrapped tampons would disappear in the fifties. Notice that despite the generally straightforward tone, tampons aren't called tampons but "in-sorbers."

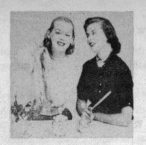

"Is Tampax really that comfortable?"

JOAN: "It certainly is! I'm not even aware I'm wearing Tampax. It's so comfortable, so convenient, that I simply couldn't ever imagine using anything else!"

PAM: "Jane told me she almost forgets about 'her time'!"

JOAN: "I do, too! Why, I'm hardly conscious of a difference in days of the month! Tampax gives so much freedom! Poise! Confidence! It's so modern. Really wonderful . . ."

PAM: (laughing) "All right! I'm sold. I'll try it this very month!"

Only by actually trying doctor-invented Tampax* internal sanitary protection, can you discover all its many advantages. Joan might have added . . . Tampax is made of surgical cotton, in disposable applicators. Easy to insert. Hands need never touch the Tampax. No chance of odor forming. It's convenient to carry "extras." Tampax comes in 3 absorbencies: Regular, Super, Junior. Sold at all drug and notion counters. Tampax Incorporated, Palmer, Mass.

* Reg. U. S. Pat. Off.

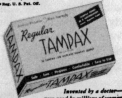

Regular TAMPAX

Invented by a doctor— now used by millions of women

By 1957, when this Tampax ad appeared in Good Housekeeping, tampons promised intangible benefits such as "poise" and "confidence." Wearing a tampon, it seemed, a woman could forget all about menstruation. The woman authority figure in the Meds ad has been replaced by a girlfriend.

claimed in ads to be "perfected by a woman doctor," but Tampax kept the upper hand with its boast of having been "invented by a doctor."

Meanwhile, the controversy in the medical community had reached the point where in April 1943, the *Western Journal of Surgery, Obstetrics & Gynecology* featured two opposing reports and an editorial on tampons. In one corner was Dr. Karl John Karnaky of Houston, who had conducted a five-year study of 42 women in which he evaluated bacteria, hydrogen ion concentration, biopsies of the vaginal mucous membrane, glycogen concentrations and "gross examination." His conclusions were overwhelmingly positive: Tampons were safe for "unmarried women"; they did not cause cancer, cervical erosion or vaginitis; they did not block menstrual flow; and they did help "the psychological attitude toward menstruation." Interestingly, Karnaky's patients used tampons not only during their periods but between periods as well, although Karnaky failed to say why or for how long. Also, two of his patients were instructed to use tampons as part of therapy to overcome sterility. Once again, no explanation was offered.[7]

In the opposite corner were the brusque Drs. J. Milton Singleton and Herbert F. Vanorden of Kansas City, who had sent questionnaires to 3,400 American and Canadian doctors. Of the 251 replies, 157 expressed "definite" opposition to tampons, while only 29 were "completely favorable." All but four strongly opposed the use of tampons by virgins, some of them noting that tampon use "created sex consciousness" and "may stimulate eroticism." Moral biases aside, 20 percent of the doctors answering the survey reported infections ranging from vaginitis to cystitis to increased menstrual cramping (dysmenorrhea), all of which they attributed directly or indirectly to tampons. "We must conclude," wrote Singleton and Vanorden, "that there is a definite potential source of infection in the habitual or occasional practice of menstrual tamponage and pre-existing infections are aggravated."[8]

The editors of the journal tried to reconcile the two views.

They expressed a dim view of "advertising propaganda and the broadcast of pseudoscientific advices," yet they acknowledged that "we are considering a subject which eludes the usual cut-and-dried manner of presentation." They observed—rather surprisingly for a medical journal—Singleton's and Vanorden's "distaste—one might almost say . . . disgust" with menstrual tampons, but they also questioned Karnaky's extolling the "absolute virtues of tampons." "Fine fuss and feathers," they concluded. Neither argument was convincing, "because to be absolutely scientific in this bracket is impossible."[9]

Impossible it may have been, but that didn't keep men and women of science from trying. The most comprehensive study to date was published by Dr. Madeline Thornton in 1943.[10] Aided by a grant from the manufacturers of Fibs tampons, she kept records on 110 women over a two-year period to see whether tampons had any harmful effects. Her conclusions: no irritations of the cervix or vagina; no new or aggravated yeast or Trichomonas infections; and no obstructions of the menstrual flow (although eight women had reported experiencing a gush of flow when they removed a tampon). Most of the women found the tampons comfortable to insert. On the negative side, only about a third of Thornton's patients felt that tampons provided complete enough protection.

Around this same time, the Personal Products Company, which manufactured Modess and Meds products (and which today is a division of Johnson & Johnson Co., and makes o.b. tampons), sponsored a sophisticated study of brand preference among what turned out to be, once again, only 25 women. This was clearly a competitive study, an attempt to prove Meds tampons superior to the industry leader, Tampax. Unlike the other four commercial tampons used in the study, and like Tampax tampons, Meds was compressed into a cardboard plunger. Although brand names aren't given in the report, published in 1944, it's not hard—by comparing the *Consumers Reports* product descriptions—to identify Meds and Tampax tampons, and it's not hard to guess which brand emerged the winner in this clinical battle. Using X-ray photographs to prove her point, the researcher—a Columbia University physician—concluded that "Tampon No. 12" (Meds) was superior because its shorter length did not deflect the cervix. The cardboard inserter was judged preferable to no inserter because of the "inevitable" contamination that resulted from manual insertion. However, it wasn't specified just what sorts of "contamination" actually occurred in the women who used inserterless tampons.[11]

Apparently Meds was also a good competitor in the drug and department stores where it was sold: The brand survived, with modifications such as a plastic inserter introduced in the late sixties, until 1977, when it finally stopped being produced.

The most entertaining—and possibly the most widely read—medical journal article on tampons appeared in the *Journal of the American Medical Association* in 1945.[12] Written by Dr. Robert Latou Dickinson (whose credits included authorship of *Human Sex Anatomy* and *Thousand Marriages*), it attempted no more than a summary of what had previously been written on the subject. What made it extraordinary were the drawings (which demonstrate that a tampon is smaller than a "phallus," and that a vagina can take any of several shapes) and the strange, condescending tone of its author:

> Month by month the "curse" hangs over one seventh of a woman's life. If strung along in sequent days, the flow would carry on for five full years. . . . Even with four pregnancies and full nursings, there are still some four hundred periods in which to use ten guards each, or some four thousand nuisances.

Dickinson took special interest in the problem of which was more erotic, napkins or tampons? The "external menstrual guard," he wrote, "is responsible for rhythmic play of pressure against surfaces uniquely alert to erotic feeling," whereas "the erotic stimulus of the stationary interior guard should be momentary and negligible . . ."

Dickinson summed up with some advice for fellow physicians when their patients asked them about tampons. If a woman is healthy and has an average flow, Dickinson wrote, she can probably wear tampons comfortably, even though she may need a sanitary napkin as well on the first day of flow. As for the future of tampons, he recommended more studies on average flow and more before-and-after examinations of tampon users.

The Dainty Years

The end of the war brought men home from the battlegrounds and into offices and factories, and it brought women home from offices and factories and into . . . home. Skirts lengthened and official morality tightened, and the feminine mystique lent a new coyness and secrecy to the menstrual products industry.

Tampax solidified its number-one position during the fifties, and held it during most of the following decade. In magazines like *Good Housekeeping*, Tampax was virtually the only brand advertised. Now the ads appeared in the front of the magazine, although they stuck to the traditional one-column, black-and-white format. Comfort and assurance were the main selling points, as illustrated in this bit of ad copy dialogue, circa 1957:

Pam: "Jane told me she almost forgets about 'her time'!"

Joan: "I do, too! Why, I'm hardly conscious of a difference in days of the month! Tampax gives so much freedom! Poise! Confidence! It's so modern. Really wonderful . . ."

The ad also notes that "hands need never touch the Tampax." The subliminal message: Menstruation is nasty—but not if you don't have to see it and touch it.

Beginning in the early fifties, Tampax also embarked on an educational program aimed at potential customers— young girls. Graphic art, brochures and speaker services helped spread the word.

Tampons were losing their aura of controversy and risk, and were starting to be regarded as harmless or even beneficial. So generally accepted did tampons become that only a handful of medical studies on their effects were published during the 1950s, and all of them concluded that tampons were innocuous, comfortable and adequate.

In fact, Dr. Karl John Karnaky, the early champion of tampons, claimed in 1956 that his 18-year study showed that tampons helped women with vaginitis! Even more amazing was his claim that tampons were a successful treatment for sterility:

> It is well known that vaginal secretions are detrimental to spermatozoa. In the study of vaginas after the removal of Tampax which had been in place for four or more hours, it has been observed many times that most of the vaginal and cervical secretion was absorbed. On artificial insemination, with and without the use of Tampax it was shown that there were more spermatozoa in the vagina when the secretions were absorbed by the tampon.[13]

I imagine that artificial insemination must have been the only alternative for these women—intercourse no doubt would have been excruciatingly painful with a tampon-dried vagina. (It is also noteworthy that here Dr. Karnaky is using "Tampax" as a generic word for tampon.)

In 1962, Dr. R. N. Rutherford and his colleagues offered still another therapeutic use for tampons: during post-delivery bleeding (lochia). Supplies of super-size tampons were donated by Tampax Incorporated. All 300 women being studied had had normal deliveries, and all began wearing tampons 10 days after delivery. Pap smears were administered three months later. At that time, 12 tampon users required cervical cauterization for healing, compared with 14 napkin users. In general, there were no significant differences between the two groups. Objections to tampons, the authors wrote, "were mainly minor and personal."[14]

Four years later, Rutherford et al endorsed tampons for "Relief of Symptomatic Vaginitis." Along with medicated creams or suppositories, the 100 patients in this study also wore tampons. Although tampons didn't make the women heal any faster, they did seem to make them more comfortable by keeping irritating discharges from reaching the sensitive lower vagina and perineum.[15]

In 1966, a team of researchers from the Rock Reproductive Clinic in Brookline, Massachusetts, published the results of their study of 903 women. They found no relationship between tampon use and abnormal conditions of the reproductive organs. But they did point out that "in order to obtain significant statistics regarding an uncommon lesion, it would be necessary to analyze thousands of cases. This would not be possible in any one institution."[16]

This particular study is interesting for another reason: It tells us that the great virginity debate was still alive and well. In a section titled "Moral and Social Considerations," the doctors from the Rock Clinic noted that it was now possible to find second-generation tampon users who began using tampons "without incident" when they started menstruating. As for the other reputed perils of tampons, they had good news: "A soft cotton tampon has no properties which would make it suitable as a dildo."

The Confidence Game

For more than ten years no new medical studies of tampons were published. It seemed as though the issue had been settled once and for all. Tampons had been proven innocuous, or even beneficial. Medical textbooks published (or revised) in the sixties and seventies praised tampons' convenience. "Certainly there are no adverse sequelae [consequences]," asserted one of the most widely read texts.[17]

Gynecologists may have lost interest in tampons, but corporate America seemed to be just discovering them. Beginning in the mid-sixties—just about the time when the medical literature falls silent—the safe, conservative menstrual products industry began undergoing some important changes.

The changes didn't seem momentous at first. In 1963, Personal Products Company had introduced Carefree, a new tampon without an applicator. It wasn't the first applicatorless tampon ever marketed—in the early days of commercial tampons many brands lacked plungers, and applicatorless Pursettes had been introduced in the early 1950s. In 1950, a European subsidiary of Personal Products' parent company, Johnson & Johnson, had introduced the applicatorless o.b. (which stands for the German *"ohne binde,"* or "without napkin"); reputedly members of the tampon industry believe that because of European women's greater willingness to touch themselves, o.b. was and is a popular brand overseas.

But for many American women, Carefree was revolutionary. It was new, its small size made it easy to carry in a purse, and it had fewer parts to be disposed of—an increasingly important concern as "ecology" crept into popular awareness. Carefree was made of rayon, not "surgical cotton" like other tampons; rayon is processed from wood pulp, making it a "natural"—although highly refined—fiber with good absorbent properties. By the seventies, rayon would supplement cotton—or supplant it—in every tampon on the market.

Carefree opened new possibilities for American women. You don't need a stiff cardboard plunger, Carefree ads implied, when your own fingers can do the job perfectly well. And even though Carefree failed to topple Tampax, it won acceptance from many women. By 1978, when *Consumer Reports* surveyed 4,500 women readers about their pref-

Wear a see-suit.
And the comfort tampon.

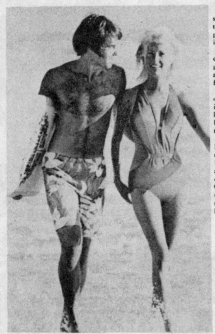

Maybe you don't know how to handle a surfboard. But why turn down the chance to wear a see-suit when the comfort tampon, Pursettes, will let you have your day in the sun?

It's the only tampon with a prelubricated tip which makes insertion easy and gentle. Pursettes doesn't even need an applicator. When you use Pursettes, you feel nothing but safe and secure.

That's because a Pursettes tampon not only fits without being felt, but because it's so protective. It's actually more absorbent than most tampons, including the leading one. Pursettes can absorb better than 10 times its own weight in fluid.

And to prove it, why not send for a free Pursettes Compact, filled with four regular Pursettes or three super-absorbent Pursettes Plus tampons. Please tell us the absorbency you prefer and enclose 25¢ to cover cost of postage-handling. Mail to Campana, Dept. SEV-970, Batavia, Ill. 60510. Then head for the ocean and ride the waves. With Pursettes, you won't know one uncomfortable moment.

Pursettes®
The only highly-absorbent tampon
with a prelubricated tip

Tampon ads abandoned coyness in the late sixties, and the swimsuit became the symbol of the freedom tampons offered. This Pursettes ad from the September 1970 issue of Seventeen took up a full page with its bold message and bright, "psychedelic" colors.

erences in menstrual products, Carefree tampons "were rated highest in overall satisfaction, protection against leakage, and wrapper disposability."[18] But Carefree never sold as well as its manufacturers would have liked, and by 1978 it was phased out in favor of o.b., which was promoted as a sophisticated European alternative. (In reality, o.b. was identical to Carefree except that it added cotton to the rayon, which probably justified a higher retail price.)

The next innovation in tampons also had modest beginnings. In 1967, International Playtex, Inc., makers of "living" brassieres and girdles, brought out a tampon with an applicator that resembled Tampax's—except that it was made out of plastic. "Soft and gentle," read a typical ad in *Seventeen*. "And its smooth, satin finish acts like a self-lubricator." The ad also boasted that Playtex was "45% more absorbent on the average than the leading tampon [Tampax]". The reason? Playtex "flowered out" (the photographs showed a dewy tulip unfolding) to fit "your inner figure." What this meant, but didn't explicitly state, was that unlike Tampax—which expanded lengthwise as it absorbed—Playtex expanded through its radius, widening instead of lengthening and therefore providing a better obstruction in the vagina.

But Playtex wasn't competing against Tampax alone. In 1970, Personal Products Company revamped its Meds tampon, and it, too, employed a plastic (polyethylene) applicator. Not only that, it had *two* withdrawal strings (for a sure grip, presumably). Meds represented an "advance" in one other important way. As a full-page *Seventeen* ad explained, Meds was made out of a new sort of material— "the most absorbent fiber ever made for a tampon"—that had taken nine years of testing on "thousands of women" to develop. The accompanying drawing showed "other" tampons' fibers magnified to look like spaghetti, while Meds' fibers looked like spaghetti strung together by cobwebs. Such was the public debut of superabsorbent fibers— chemically manipulated cotton or rayon that expands many-fold when exposed to moisture, like one of those wafer-thin sponges that instantly grow to full size when dropped in a dishpan. (See Chapter 1 for a fuller explanation of super-absorbents.)

Playtex, a newcomer in the "feminine hygiene" business, managed to hold its own, but barely, against these formidable industry giants. But the marketing men at Playtex knew women—or thought they did. Their next move was, in marketing terms, a brilliant and inventive one. It was responsible for catapulting Playtex into a major position in the tampon industry, and it had a lasting effect on the way all tampons were advertised.

The secret was smell. Playtex decided that women thought their menstrual fluid had an unpleasant odor, and Playtex came up with a solution: "deodorant" tampons. In fact, there was no deodorant in Playtex tampons—only a heavy, cloying fragrance (which in the ads was called a "fresh, delicate scent"). The product was introduced in 1971 with a small-type warning label on boxes, cautioning women to see their doctors "if sensitivity or irritation occurs." Many women did: They had developed allergic reactions to the fragrance. Although Playtex insisted—and still insists—that its perfume is "totally safe," according to Playtex's director of consumer affairs, Leonard Berger, the company quietly picked up the medical bills of women who complained. Privately, Playtex pooh-poohed the complaints. "Women had problems before tampons were ever invented," one Playtex executive told me.

It was a classic case of "create a need and fill it," and the Playtex advertising campaigns harped obsessively on themes of worry, security and detection. One 1972 magazine ad featured a woman at a party, looking at the camera with an expression of distress. "When you're wearing a tampon you don't worry about odor," the copy read. "But should you?" The implication was that yes, you certainly should. The irony was that no, you certainly shouldn't. Menstrual fluid has no odor until it's exposed to air, which doesn't happen with *any* tampon until it's removed. Still, the late sixties and early seventies were a heyday for genital scents; flavored douches and vaginal sprays were targeted at the "love generation," which seemingly didn't love its own natural odors. Deodorant tampons were a hit despite common sense and physiological reality—and despite the fact that doctors were becoming increasingly alarmed by the vaginal irritations caused by the fragrance, and were beginning to advise their patients not to use the tampons.

Playtex deodorant (and nondeodorant) tampons were aided enormously by a major marketing breakthrough. In 1972, the National Association of Broadcasters, a TV industry self-regulatory body, lifted a ban on TV advertising of sanitary napkins, tampons and douche products. "Lack of audience resistance" to the ads when they had been shown on non-code stations was given as the reason. The response on the part of some tampon manufacturers was slow at first—Tampax refused to advertise on TV until 1978—but they soon made up for their early reluctance with commercials depicting well-groomed women discussing their intimate physiological functions with unsettling candor. Annual expenditures for tampon advertising on TV doubled between 1975 and 1978, with serious consequences for Tampax: The industry leader's market share fell from 90 percent to about 70 percent of what was by then a $136 million-a-year field.[19]

The race was on. Tampon companies used sophisticated psychological ploys, capitalizing on women's doubts about their bodies' natural functions and odors, to sell their products. "Trust," "security" and "confidence" were the lures. "I didn't trust o.b., than I saw how those layers protected against leaks," confided one two-page ad. Pursettes, "the comfort tampon," was said to "end worrying." Magazine advertising became graphic, with photographs of tampons expanded in beakers of water, or with, even, anatomical drawings. The tactics worked well: By 1980, 70 percent of American women used tampons at some time.[20] For many women, apparently convinced by the ads, tampon use wasn't even restricted to menstrual periods: These women were wearing the new tampons between their periods so that they'd feel even more "secure."

The most spectacular use of the confidence bait—indeed, the most sensational story in the history of the tampon industry—was the campaign for Rely tampons. Rely was the first "feminine hygiene product" ever manufactured by giant Procter & Gamble ($10.82 billion in corporate sales in 1980), makers of household and personal products like Crest, Tide and Ivory, and the number-one advertiser in the United States. P&G threw all of its considerable corporate weight behind Rely research, development and marketing. Development began in 1962, but the new tampon wasn't even test-marketed until 1974, in Fort Wayne, Indiana. That debut was quickly followed by test markets in Rochester, New York (1975), Kansas City (1977) and Seattle and Portland, Oregon (1978). National marketing followed in 1980.

The product's name was a virtual command to women to put their faith in it. "It even absorbs the worry," Rely's slogan, told women what, presumably, they wanted to hear: that there would never be a trace of leakage to betray their secret.

The trick was in Rely's radically different design. Instead of being made of compressed fibers, Rely consisted of tiny polyester sponges and confetti-like chips of carboxymethylcellulose, a chemically modified cellulose, all loosely wrapped inside a polyester sac. The whole thing was encased in an opaque plastic inserter whose "petal" tip opened upon insertion to form four sharp cusps. Folded inside the applicator, the tampon seemed small, but upon exposure to liquid it instantly expanded to two or three times its original volume. The innovative design, P&G executives explained, was a response to women's complaints that their tampons didn't offer enough protection against leaks during a heavy flow. Just how real those "heavy flows" were is a matter for conjecture. It's been suggested that when large numbers of women stopped taking birth control pills in the seventies, their menstrual flows readjusted from the artificially light conditions under the Pill. Now that they were flowing normally again, some of these women perceived the amount of blood as abnormally large, compared to when they were on the Pill.[21] Tampon manufacturers didn't enlighten them.

With Rely, Procter & Gamble broke new ground. In the spring of 1980, when the tampon was introduced nationally, P&G spent $10 million to distribute free samples of Rely tampons to 80 percent of the nation's households. The previous year—before Rely was out of test market—the company had spent $7.8 million on advertising. As a result, Rely skyrocketed in popularity, grabbing 17 percent of sales and becoming the nation's number-three selling brand virtually overnight. (Tampax still led the pack with 42 percent of the market, while Playtex held on to second place with 25 percent.)

But there were problems from the start. In Rochester, the Empire State Consumer Association raised questions about one of Rely's original ingredients, polyurethane. Polyurethane foam is used in many industrial applications, including insulation. And it has been found to be carcinogenic when implanted in animals. A number of Rochester women—who apparently weren't aware that they were "guinea pigs" in a test market—had complaints about Rely. "It felt like trying to remove an opened-up umbrella," one woman told the Rochester *Patriot*. Others complained that the tampons broke apart during use or caused vaginal itching and burning. P&G sent company representatives to meet with the group, and in the end agreed to reformulate the tampon, leaving out polyurethane.

But suspicions remained, and the time was right for consumers to start questioning the products they used. Beginning around the mid-seventies, women involved in the feminist health-care movement began taking a critical look at all tampons. Deodorant tampons were obvious targets for scrutiny, since scented douches and vaginal sprays had recently come under attack. But what else was in tampons? Women suddenly realized that they didn't know.

Nor would tampon manufacturers tell them. When concerned women wrote to the companies, they were told that the contents of tampons were "proprietary information." Angry and frustrated, women in some feminist health clinics began publicizing some of their own suspicions about tampons, alleging that they contained harmful additives such as asbestos or chemicals that caused more bleeding; that they were packaged wastefully; and that they could be too absorbent and drying in a normal vagina.

Acting as individuals or as small, frequently impoverished collectives, these women couldn't possibly sponsor the kind of research it would take to prove their charges. So it wasn't until women with actual tampon damage began showing up in clinics that the medical establishment started—slowly—paying attention to tampons again.

The first warnings came in 1977. Writing in the *American Journal of Obstetrics and Gynecology*, a team of Colorado researchers reported on four cases of "tampon-induced vaginal or cervical ulceration."[22] All of the cases were women who used tampons chronically to absorb persistent vaginal "drainage." One of the patients had used tampons continuously for four and a half months; another had used deodorized tampons "intermittently and chronically" for seven months. Two were adolescent virgins. All had visible ulcers on their cervixes or vaginas and all healed when they stopped using tampons. The authors theorized that the ulcers may have been caused by the pressure of tampons against sensitive tissue, or by "an idiosyncratic reaction to the chemicals in the deodorized tampons."

Few gynecologists probably read the next ominous report on tampons, which appeared in the *Journal of Family Practice* in 1979.[23] In it, a Mississippi family practitioner described a single case of heavy vaginal bleeding caused by a plastic tampon inserter. The patient, a 21-year-old woman, had apparently "been in a hurry when she inserted her first tampon," and arterial laceration had resulted from a plastic cusp on the end of her inserter. (The tampon brand was not named, but only Playtex was at this time marketing tampons with plastic, petal-shaped inserters in Mississippi.) The physician concluded: "This patient had a life-threatening hemorrhage from a small laceration brought on by the careless insertion of a tampon."

By this time nearly every tampon on the market used some type of modified superabsorbent cellulose. All of the companies claim that, before they reformulated, they conducted laboratory and clinical tests to make sure their products were safe. However, none of this research surfaced in the medical journals until 1980, when two alarming reports were published in *Obstetrics & Gynecology*, the official journal of the American College of Obstetricians and Gynecologists, which claims some 25,000 doctor members.

The first article, written by Drs. Eduard G. Friedrich, Jr. and Kenneth A. Siegesmund from the University of Wisconsin, was sponsored by a grant from Kimberly-Clark Corporation (headquartered in Neenah, Wisconsin).[24] By now, Kimberly-Clark was manufacturing, in addition to an extensive line of sanitary napkins and mini- and maxi-pads, Kotex Stick Tampons and (in some parts of the country) Kotex Security Tampons. Both used superabsorbent fibers; the stick tampons were made with "Supercotton" and the security tampons (which have plastic inserters) with "Ultrasorb" and two other, unnamed, fibers. Obviously, Kimberly-Clark had high stakes in the controlled study it sponsored to assess "the acute effects of tampon exposure."

One hundred and sixty women gave their informed consent to participate in the study. They were divided into two groups of 80; one group wore tampons during their menstrual periods, and the other group wore tampons between their periods. "Three of the leading brands" were used; none contained fragrance. Each woman received either "conventional" tampons, or "superabsorbent" tampons of the same brand, or no tampons (the control group). The study was both random and "blind," meaning the doctors doing the study didn't know which tampon brand the women received. Each woman was examined with a colposcope—an instrument that allows the doctor to examine the vagina and cervix under low power magnification—either between or during menses, depending on when she was using the tampons.

What Friedrich and Siegesmund found was that although the brand of tampon made no difference—all three produced alterations of the mucosa—superabsorbency made a big difference. In each group of 80, 13 women developed microulcerations—microscopically visible sores—in the vaginal mucous membrane. Ten out of each group of 13 had been using "supers." In addition, among women who used "supers" there were many cases of dryness and layering of the membrane cells; several of these changes occurred after only two hours of tampon use. All abnormalities cleared up within a month after tampon use stopped.

These were alarming findings for, as the authors noted, "vaginal ulcerations are uncommon lesions." They concluded that superabsorbent cellulose tampons were responsible for these lesions, especially in women who used them between periods for "spotting" caused by the birth control pill or "to absorb what they perceive to be an abnormal amount of vaginal secretion."

Friedrich and Siegesmund did not presume to advise against the use of superabsorbent tampons, although that implication seemed clear. In any event, what they—and the women they studied—probably didn't know was that many of the "conventional" tampons they used were made of superabsorbent fibers—just fewer of them, so that their overall bulk was smaller.

Meanwhile, clinical cases were accumulating in gynecologists' offices. At the Mary Imogene Bassett Hospital in Cooperstown, New York, gynecologists were baffled by the sudden appearance of the first cases of tampon-associated ulcers any of them had ever seen—seven cases since early 1979. These were not microulcerations; they were large sores visible under low-power magnification or even with the naked eye. As the chief of the hospital's ob-gyn department told an FDA panel hearing in October 1980, "These are terrible-looking ulcers." The doctors' first concern was that they might be cancerous. They weren't—in fact, they all cleared up quickly and easily—but that didn't make them any less frightening.

At the same FDA hearing, Dr. Ken Noller, a gynecologist from the Mayo Clinic, warned those in attendance that he was going to show slides of some of these "awful" ulcers. "Any of you who . . . get a bit squeamish by seeing blood and things like that," he cautioned, "had best leave." His slides revealed not only ulcers but bits of tampon fiber embedded in them. Neither physician was able to offer a definitive explanation of how tampons caused ulcers, what the consequences of untreated ulcers might be, or why the ulcers disappeared so quickly with treatment and abstinence from tampons. Even more mysterious was the fact that the women who had the ulcers did not report any symptoms related to them; all had come into the clinics for routine examinations or because of some unrelated gynecological problem. Because of this, the two doctors at the hearing agreed that they were probably seeing only a tiny fraction of the ulcers actually represented in the tampon-wearing population.

Evidence of tampon-induced damage continued to mount. In the July 1980 issue of *Obstetrics & Gynecology*, two Oklahoma physicians described 10 cases of vaginal ulcers resulting from the use of synthetic-fiber tampons.[25] In this report, brands were named—Tampax, Kotex, Playtex and Rely—but "super" and "regular" types were not differentiated. The patients had all used tampons continuously for nonmenstrual reasons; one had used them for six months. All of the lesions (with one exception) healed when tampon use was discontinued. Although some cases also required treatment with antibiotic creams, one case required surgery.

Clearly, these were developments of a serious and surprising nature, developments that demanded further study and the cooperation of doctors in educating their patients about tampon use. But by July 1980, the reports of ulcerations and lacerations had been dramatically eclipsed by a strange new disease that seemed to strike down young women—and in some cases kill them—at the peak of their womanhood, during active menstruation. The disease was

called toxic shock syndrome, and the suspected cause—
direct or indirect—was tampons.

NOTES

1. Lloyd Arnold and Marie Hagele, "Vaginal Tamponage for Catamenial Sanitary Protection," *Journal of the American Medical
   Association* 110:790, March 1938.

2. *British Medical Journal*, 2:1113; (November 26, 1938) 2 (December 17, 1938):1282; 1 (January 7, 1939):36.

3. "Sanitary Pads and Tampons," *Consumers Reports*, June 1942,
   pp. 157–60.

4. Maurice O. Magid and Jacob Geiger, "The Intravaginal Tampon
   in Menstrual Hygiene: A Clinical Study," *Medical Record* 155
   (May 1942):316.

5. Sune Genell and Anders Lysander, "Några fall av skadegörelse
   genom 'Tampax'" (Some cases of injury from "Tampax"), *Sven-
   ska Läkartidniningen* 36 (December 8, 1939):2236–2240.

6. Mary Barton, "Review of the Sanitary Appliance With a Discussion on Intravaginal Packs," *British Medical Journal* 1 (April 25,
   1942):524.

7. Karl John Karnaky, "Vaginal Tampons for Menstrual Hygiene,"
   Western Journal of Surgery, Obstetrics & Gynecology 51 (April
   1943):146.

8. J. Milton Singleton and Herbert F. Vanorden, "Vaginal Tampons
   in Menstrual Hygiene," *ibid*; p. 146.

9. "Intravaginal Menstrual 'Hygiene,'" *ibid*; p. 171.

10. Madeline J. Thornton, "Use of Vaginal Tampons for the Ab-
    sorption of Menstrual Discharges," *American Journal of Obstet-
    rics and Gynecology* 46 (August 1943):259.

11. Irja Elizabeth Widenius, "A Study of Commercially Manufactured
    Catamenial Tampons," *American Journal of Obstetrics and Gyne-
    cology* 48 (October 1944):510.

12. Robert Latou Dickinson, "Tampons as Menstrual Guards," *Jour-
    nal of the American Medical Association* 128 (June 16, 1945):490.

13. Karl John Karnaky, "Vaginal Tampons for Menstrual Hygiene: Second Report—An 18-Year Study," *Clinical Medicine* 3 (June 1956):545.

14. R. N. Rutherford, A. Lawrence Banks and W. A. Coburn, "Intravaginal Tampons for the Postpartum Patient," *Obstetrics and Gynecology* 19:781 June 1962.

15. Rutherford, Banks and Coburn, "Tampons in Relief of Symptomatic Vaginitis," *Pacific Medicine and Surgery* 74:314, November–December 1966.

16. Robert E. Wheatley, Miriam F. Menkin, Eleanor Dooks Bardes and John Rock, "Tampons in Menstrual Hygiene," *Journal of the American Medical Association* 192:697 May 24, 1965.

17. Edmund R. Novak, Georgeanna Seegar Jones and Howard W. Jones, *Novak's Textbook of Gynecology,* 8th ed., (Baltimore: Williams & Wilkins, 1970), p. 78.

18. "Menstrual Tampons and Pads," *Consumer Reports*, March 1978, p. 127.

19. "Tampax faces life," *Forbes*, May 29, 1978, p. 61.

20. "Toxic-Shock Syndrome—United States, 1970–1980" *Morbidity and Mortality Weekly Report*, January, 30, 1981, Vol. 30, p. 27.

21. Cynthia W. Cooke and Susan Dworkin, "The Tempered Tampon," *Ms.*, December 1980, p. 64.

22. Kathryn F. Barrett, Sonia Bledsoe, Benjamin E. Greer and William Droegemueller, "Tampon-induced Vaginal or Cervical Ulceration," *American Journal of Obstetrics and Gynecology* 127:332, February 1, 1977.

23. Robert K. Collins, "Tampon-Induced Vaginal Laceration," *The Journal of Family Practice* 9:127, July 1979.

24. Eduard G. Friedrich, Jr. and Kenneth A. Siegesmund, "Tampon-Associated Vaginal Ulcerations," *Obstetrics and Gynecology* 55:149, February 1980.

25. Steven D. Jimerson and John D. Becker, "Vaginal Ulcers Associated with Tampon Usage," *Obstetrics and Gynecology* 56:97, July 1980.

CHAPTER 4

Toxic Shock Syndrome

The Mystery Disease

To Dr. Joan Chesney, chief of the pediatrics infectious disease division at the University of Wisconsin School of Medicine, "It was like being hit over the head with a sledgehammer."

Chesney's husband Russell, a nephrologist (kidney specialist) at the medical school, had come home on December 1, 1979, with news about a puzzling case. A 18-year-old woman had been admitted to the hospital with kidney failure and had been diagnosed as having hemolytic-uremic syndrome—a kidney disease whose cause is unknown. "But there's something wrong," Russell Chesney kept saying. "It just isn't typical." For one thing, the young woman had a high fever and was in shock—unusual in cases of this kidney disease. She also had muscle aches, red eyes reminiscent of conjunctivitis, and a sunburn-like rash, none of which usually accompany hemolytic-uremic syndrome. Finally, her illness had struck with sudden force over the course of a single day; it generally takes about a week for hemolytic-uremic syndrome patients to become seriously ill.

As her husband described the case, Joan Chesney remembered an article she'd read in the British medical journal *The Lancet* just a year earlier. The article, by Denver pediatrician James Todd, two other pediatricians and a microbiologist, identified a new disease called toxic shock syndrome in seven children between the ages of 8 and 17.[1] Its symptoms included high fever, sore throat, headache, watery diarrhea, low blood pressure that sometimes led to shock, a bright red rash, and kidney and liver failure; its cause was thought to be a toxin (poison) produced by a bacterium, Staphylococcus aureus, that's commonly found on the skin. Its consequences could be tragic: One of Todd's patients died, and another developed gangrene as a result of shock. Could Russell Chesney's patient be suffering from toxic shock syndrome?

A few days later, as the kidney patient gradually recovered, Joan Chesney had two more opportunities to test her hypothesis. At noon on December 5, a 15-year-old girl was brought to Madison General Hospital in shock. Her other symptoms matched Todd's description of toxic shock syndrome. Alarmed by the severity of her condition, the pediatrics residents came down to Joan Chesney's office to tell her about the case. The girl's private physician had accompanied her to the hospital, and he was "distraught," Chesney remembers. "He told us that she'd been in the hospital a month before, to the day, with very similar— although milder—symptoms." Russell Chesney's kidney patient also had had symptoms of her illness the previous month.

The same day, Joan Chesney heard about a third case with the same baffling symptoms. A 25-year-old woman had been admitted to Madison General on December 3; the tentative diagnosis was kidney infection with shock, but her doctors hadn't been able to find a cause. They gave her supportive treatment—consisting mostly of intravenous fluids—and on December 5, they presented her case to a joint pediatrics and adult infectious disease conference at the hospital. Joan Chesney hadn't planned to attend the conference, but at the last minute she decided to go. As she listened to the description of this new case, she suddenly realized that it fit Todd's description of toxic shock syndrome once again, this time in an adult. It was a remarkable cluster of cases that defied coincidence. "It looked like an outbreak," Chesney says.

As soon as the conference ended, Joan and Russell Chesney called Dr. Jeff Davis, Wisconsin's state epidemiologist. (Epidemiology is the study of the origin and distribution of diseases.) Like the Chesneys, Davis was aware of the work of James Todd in Denver. He knew that Todd's seven cases had occurred over a period of two and a half years. Now, in Madison, there had been three cases within just four days, all of them fitting Todd's description of the disease's symptoms. "It was very unusual," Davis observes. "I immediately got intensively involved."

The first thing he did was to come to Madison and interview the Chesneys' three patients to find out what they had in common besides being young women from the west side of Madison. During Davis's conversation with one of the teenage patients, he discovered a piece of information that hadn't been on the young woman's chart: She had been menstruating on the day she fell ill. Davis quickly asked the other patients about their menstrual histories and found out that they, too, had been having their periods when they became ill. Once again, it seemed to be more than coincidence.

In the next few weeks, Joan Chesney heard about two women in Wisconsin who'd had toxic shock syndrome symptoms over the past summer. And in January, two more patients entered Madison hospitals with the now-familiar high fever, nausea and vomiting, sunburn-like rash and low blood pressure. One of these new patients was a young girl who hadn't yet started menstruating; in her case, the Staphylococcus infection seemed to stem from abscesses on her heels. But the other patient was a young woman who was menstruating when she suddenly became severely ill.

Then, around the middle of January, Dr. Davis received a phone call from Dr. Andrew Dean, Davis's counterpart in the Minnesota Department of Health. Dean told Davis about five recent cases of "something pretty frightening." It was toxic shock syndrome, and it was hitting young women. "We think it has something to do with menses" was all Davis could say at the time. The Minnesota cases, added to the Wisconsin cases, made 12 recent documented cases of toxic shock syndrome. All anyone could do for the patients was give them plenty of intravenous fluids and hope that out of a battery of antibiotics, one might ease the condition.

Davis and Dean agreed that it was time to report the cases to the federal Centers for Disease Control in Atlanta, an agency that counts and studies outbreaks of infectious disease. Davis took one additional step to alert the public to toxic shock syndrome. On January 31, he sent a letter to 3,500 internists, family practitioners and pediatricians in Wisconsin. The letter described the original cases cited by Dr. Todd, the symptoms of toxic shock syndrome, its newfound association with menses, and its possible association with Staphylococcus aureus. The last piece of information let doctors know that anti-staphylococcal drugs should be considered for treatment. The response to the letter was startling. "We started getting cases reported to us almost immediately," says Davis.

A Milwaukee doctor received the letter while one of her young patients was in the hospital with undiagnosed symptoms. The doctor realized, after reading Davis's letter, that the girl had toxic shock syndrome. She told the girl's parents that their daughter might be suffering from a new disease. Alarmed, the parents mentioned the "new disease" to some neighbors, who in turn called the Milwaukee *Journal*. On Valentine's Day 1980, the *Journal* published the first newspaper account of toxic shock syndrome—or TSS, as it was beginning to be called. The story included Dr. Davis's office telephone number so that doctors and women who thought they'd had the disease could call in their reports.

"We had a *lot* of calls," Davis says. "Not every woman who called had had TSS—but many of them had. It was a very effective surveillance system in that it allowed us to learn about a lot of cases in a short period of time."

Next, Davis and his co-workers began the task of finding out what had caused all these young women to become so sick so quickly. They developed a study not only of women who'd had TSS but of a control group—women of the same ages and menstrual histories who hadn't become ill. All told, there were 35 cases and 105 controls, and between March and May they were interviewed about a wide range of factors—exercise patterns, vaginal infections, sexual contact, contraception, and type of menstrual product used.

Davis had had a hunch, early on, that tampons might have something to do with TSS in menstruating women, if only because they were "an internal device." As it turned out, the numbers supported his hunch: Out of 35 cases, 34 had been using tampons when they became ill, a rate of 97 percent. By contrast, 80 out of 105 controls—76 percent—used tampons during every menstrual period.[2] Why the correlation? Nobody could explain it.

The Wisconsin team learned a few other things about TSS. Nearly a third of the menstruating women who'd gotten the disease had more than one episode, all during menses; five women had three or more recurrences. But patients who'd been treated with a certain family of drugs called beta-lactamase-resistant antibiotics had significantly fewer recurrences than women who'd been treated with antibiotics such as penicillin and ampicillin. The researchers also discovered that a smaller percentage of TSS victims than controls had been using any method of birth control; this may or may not have been significant, given the fact that most of the women who'd had TSS were quite young (12 in the study were 18 or younger).

By the time the Wisconsin study was nearing completion, the Centers for Disease Control (CDC) published their first report of what was shaping up as a nationwide outbreak of the new disease. On May 23, the centers' *Morbidity and Mortality Weekly Report*, sent free to anyone who requests it (see Appendix), told of 55 cases reported by state health departments in Wisconsin, Minnesota, Illinois, Utah and Idaho, and by physicians in eight other states. Among the 55 cases were seven deaths.

Almost overnight, the story of toxic shock syndrome was on front pages of newspapers around the country. Throughout the summer of 1980, as the number of reported TSS cases kept climbing, it seemed as though you couldn't turn on the television or radio, or pick up a newspaper or magazine, without noticing a report about the mysterious new disease that struck down healthy young women in the middle of a normal, essential body process: menstruation.

The Suspect Tampon

Although by the summer it was generally agreed that tampons had *something* to do with TSS, no one knew exactly what or why. And no one had yet shown that certain brands or types of tampons were more likely to be associated with the disease than others. "As far as I could tell," admits Dr. Davis, "there wasn't much known about tampons at all."

While researchers from the CDC were interviewing women who'd had TSS about the brand and type of tampons they'd used, some TSS victims took matters in their own hands. They knew that tampons had caused their disease, these women said, and they were holding tampon manufacturers responsible. Tampons had changed over the last few years, they charged, but tampon makers hadn't let women know. They speculated that the changes in tampons may well have created the perfect environment for the bug that caused TSS.

The first company to be sued was Procter & Gamble, makers of Rely. Linda Imboden, a 27-year-old home health-aide and mother of three children from the town of Redding in northern California, had had a severe case of TSS in May 1980. She'd thought she was coming down with the flu until her blood pressure plummeted to 48/0; as a result of the loss of circulation, a third of her hair fell out and gangrene destroyed the tips of eight fingers and three toes, some of which had to be amputated. Four months after she was hospitalized, she still suffered muscle aches.

Linda Imboden had used Rely tampons for about a year, ever since she'd received a free sample in the mail. "I liked them at first," she told me. "There was less leakage." But in August 1980 she decided to sue Procter & Gamble for $5 million in punitive damages, alleging that the company had known six months earlier that there were serious problems related to Rely.

Soon she was joined by other TSS victims—and not just Rely users—in claiming that tampon makers had shown negligence in not warning women about the risks associated with tampons. In October, a Los Angeles woman, 30-year-old Lynette Edelson, sued Johnson & Johnson, makers of o.b. tampons. Edelson, the mother of two children, had come down with TSS in January 1980; she'd had a temperature of 104 degrees, had been hospitalized for six days, and hadn't expected to live. "Until articles came out about TSS, I thought I had some very strange disease," she told a newspaper reporter. Her suit asked for $2 million in damages. Another 30-year-old Los Angeles woman, Cheryl Schwartz, had spent two weeks in an intensive care unit in the fall of 1979 while doctors puzzled over her 105-degree fever, rash, diarrhea and general debilitation. When she finally got better—she still suffers some mild symptoms—she set about researching her disease. In September she filed a $10 million suit against International Playtex, makers of the Playtex tampon she'd been wearing when she became ill.

In all, every tampon manufacturer except Purex (makers of Pursettes) has been sued by at least one TSS victim. By the end of 1980, the total number of lawsuits filed against tampon makers had reached 15, including 4 class action suits.

But the tampon that got most of the blame was Rely. Rely was different, women insisted—just look at it. It wasn't the familiar compressed fiber cylinder but a polyester bag loosely filled with foam and tiny chips of a strange substance that swelled and turned gel-like when they were wet. Some women had noticed that Rely was difficult to remove—it seemed to "scrape" the vaginal walls. And nobody had heard of TSS before Rely was introduced. Wasn't that enough of a connection?

It was one of those instances when intuition is borne out—if not by science, then by statistics. In September 1980 the CDC released the results of a follow-up study of 50 selected TSS cases.[3] Among the women who'd used only one brand of tampon during the menstrual period when they became ill, 71 percent—nearly three quarters—had used Rely. That the remaining women had used all of the other major tampon brands tended to get glossed over in the uproar that ensued. Some stores began immediately removing packages of Rely from displays. And within a week of the CDC report, Procter & Gamble decided to cut its losses. Although company officials insisted (and continue to insist) that they knew of "no defect" in Rely, they chose to remove the tampon from the market and to offer refunds to women who had used or unused packages at home. The move was expected to cost Procter & Gamble $75 million.

The Search for a Cause

Meanwhile, the cases accumulated—941 by January 1981, including 73 deaths. Nine hundred five of the reported cases had been menstruating women. But as the novelty of the syndrome's association with menstrution wore off, more unusual cases began being reported—TSS in men, in menopausal women, in women who'd just delivered babies.

In the laboratories and offices of the Centers for Disease Control, scientists tried to figure out how and why toxic shock syndrome attacked the largest risk group—young, menstruating women. What did the victims have in common besides the fact that almost all of them used tampons? What about tampons enhanced the growth of the bacteria or its toxins? Could a specific toxin be identified as the cause of the syndrome? Was an antitoxin on the horizon?

Although clues have appeared and breakthroughs promised, these questions remain largely unanswered. But the following provocative theories have been advanced:

• *Any tampon, if left in the vagina long enough, becomes a breeding ground for bacteria.*

This is a commonsense observation that offers only a partial explanation. It's true that bacteria love to feast on blood—the preferred medium for growing bacteria in laboratories is blood agar. Some doctors leaped to the conclusion that tampons ought to be changed frequently to prevent bacteria from growing; the American College of Obstetrics and Gynecology even published a recommendation to that effect. And early results from a study (as yet unpublished) done by the state health departments of Iowa, Minnesota and Wisconsin indicate that the onset of TSS tends to cluster around the early morning hours, after the women have worn tampons all night. But many women who use tampons at night *don't* become ill. Why wearing time seems to be a factor for some women and not others is still unknown.

• *Synthetic tampons scratch the vaginal membranes, providing a route into the bloodstream for Staphylococcus aureus toxins.*

This theory combines recent observations about a relationship between synthetic, superabsorbent tampons and vaginal ulcers with observations about TSS. It was proposed by several physicians who'd seen a few TSS cases and a few ulceration cases, but it's been challenged by other researchers—notably James Todd, the doctor who coined the term "toxic shock syndrome," and Patrick Schlievert, a

University of Minnesota microbiologist who has been studying S. aureus and its toxins since 1978. Schlievert says that although vaginal ulcers may be breeding grounds for S. aureus, the toxin produced by that bacterium passes easily through membranes without benefit of a break in the tissue. One of the problems with testing any theory about ulcers and TSS is that few TSS patients have been examined with a colposcope (an instrument that permits low-power magnification of the cells of the vagina and cervix) during their illness, and tampon-caused ulcers tend to heal rather quickly.

• *Something about Rely made it more likely to cause TSS than any other tampon.*

This commonsense theory hasn't checked out so far. CDC researchers haven't been able to culture Staphylococcus aureus from any commercial tampon. And nothing in Rely's contents has been shown to enhance the growth of S. aureus toxins. Yet the CDC in January 1981 pointed to an apparent decline in TSS cases, and inferred that Rely's recall was responsible in part.[4] This claim was challenged by public health officials in Iowa, Minnesota and Wisconsin, who say that the decline was more a matter of a lack of active surveillance, and that all tampon brands were still associated with TSS. But even the tristate researchers acknowledged in their study "some indication of increased risk associated with Rely brand tampons beyond that predicted by their absorbency." The reason? It's still a mystery.

• *The more absorbent a tampon, the greater the risk of TSS.*

That's the conclusion reached by the tristate study. This study looked at 80 women who'd had TSS and 160 who hadn't. The researchers determined levels of tampon absorbency using data supplied by the tampon industry—data from clinical trials as well as from laboratory tests with a synthetic vagina that mimicked the pressure inside a human vagina. They found that although, within each brand, "super" tampons absorbed more than "regular" ones, some brands' "regulars" were as absorbent as other brands' "supers." And women who used the higher absorbency tampons had a 17 to 30 times greater risk of getting TSS, while those who used the least absorbent tampons had only two to three times the risk of a woman who didn't use tampons at all.

The CDC will not confirm these findings—but, as Minnesota state epidemiologist Dr. Michael Osterholm points out, the CDC *can't*. Its only study, conducted in the summer of 1980, included only 15 women, and the absorbency of the brands they used was never ascertained.

• *Tampons dam up the menstrual blood, causing it to back up into the uterus and out the fallopian tubes, where any toxins in it may be absorbed in the abdominal cavity.*

This theory of "retrograde" (backwards) menstrual flow was proposed by four doctors at Massachusetts General Hospital.[6] In the 1930s and 40s, researchers had decided that tampons did *not* cause the menstrual flow to back up. However, the Massachusetts doctors observed that tampons had changed since those years, and that "newly introduced devices have been designed to expand several fold and occlude [block] the vaginal outlet." Their hypothesis is tantalizing yet difficult to prove, and so far no one has attempted to do so.

• *Something besides tampons—perhaps something associated with menses itself—is responsible for TSS in menstruating women.*

This is the "tampon-as-red-herring" theory. Proponents point out that 70 percent of American women use tampons, yet only .003 to .015 percent seem to be getting TSS. Perhaps, this theory goes, tampons are a statistical cofactor, not a biological one, and something else is going on in the vaginas of the women who become ill.

Obviously, this theory is favored by tampon makers. But it's also attractive to some researchers. Dr. Shirley Fannin, chief of acute communicable disease control for Los Angeles County, says that tampons must not be a high-risk factor in TSS if so many women use them and so few women get TSS. "At most," she says, "tampons may be a cofactor— or possibly an enhancer—in the growth of the Staphylococcus aureus toxin. Why couldn't one say that *menstruation* is the common biological factor in the disease?"

Supporting this theory is the fact that many women's immunological resistance is low just before and during menstruation. Certain skin ailments—from pimples to herpes—are more common around the menstrual period. Since Staphylococcus is associated with many diseases involving rashes, boils and other skin symptoms, there may indeed be a clue here. However, menstruation, like many other normal body functions, hasn't been studied thoroughly enough for scientists to say with authority just what that clue might point to.

Putting TSS in Perspective

Toxic shock syndrome may be just one member of a class of diseases caused by Staphylococcus aureus. For example, there's a type of "scarlet fever" that causes milder forms of the characteristic TSS symptoms: fever, rash, muscle aches. Although classic scarlet fever is associated with Streptococcus bacteria, this similar illness is caused by Staphylococcus, and is called "scalded-skin syndrome."

Somewhat more severe, but also caused by Staphylococcus aureus toxin, is Kawasaki's disease (also called mucocutaneous lymph node syndrome). It involves conjunctivitis ("pink eye") and peeling as well as fever. It was first reported around 1975—the same year James Todd began seeing TSS cases in children in Colorado—by a Japanese pediatrician, Tomisaku Kawasaki. More than 10,000 cases of Kawasaki's disease have been diagnosed in Japan, mostly in infants. One of those infants even developed gangrenous fingers, just like some women who've had TSS. And articles published in 1979 and 1980 in American medical journals described several cases of Kawasaki's disease in adults. In fact, when Patrick Schlievert first began studying TSS, he called it "adult Kawasaki's disease."

Part of the problem in tracing the history of TSS is the frequency with which it's misdiagnosed. Before the CDC made its first report on TSS, patients with all the classic symptoms were told they had everything from flu to meningitis to kidney infection. It's possible that many past cases of TSS are hidden under incorrect labels.

And some TSS cases may be hiding even now. The CDC's case definition for the disease is very strict: A victim must have a fever of at least 102 degrees, rash, peeling within two weeks after the onset of illness, very low blood pressure (less than 90 mm Hg for adults), and involvement of three or more organ systems. But many women who've been severely ill lacked one or more of these symptoms. For example, some patients died before peeling had started; these cases are described only as "probable" by the CDC. Still other cases appear to be mild versions of TSS.

Most doctors and researchers agree that it's possible to experience a mild form of TSS, but only in Wisconsin and Minnesota are public health officials actively seeking reports of mild cases. "We don't use them epidemiologically," explains Dr. Jeff Davis of the Wisconsin Division of Health. "But we do recognize them. Not everyone has shock. Not everyone is severely ill. We have to realize that not everyone will have the same form of the disease."

What's Being Done About TSS?

The effort to find answers to questions about TSS continues on many fronts. In fact, at this writing some researchers are expecting major breakthroughs within a matter of months.

At the Centers for Disease Control, researchers are looking into factors *other* than tampons that are associated with

TSS. Why, for example, does TSS seem to strike young white women more than other age and racial groups? (In Los Angeles County, where about a third of the population is Hispanic, all but three of the TSS cases on record as of March 1981 were in non-Spanish-surname Caucasian women.) CDC researchers have been unable to culture S. aureus from any commercial tampon; how, then, does the bacterium find its way into the vagina? Does it live in the external genital skin and become introduced into the vagina when a tampon (or a finger) is introduced? Or is there some other explanation? Why haven't there been the same proportion of TSS cases in Canada and Europe as there have been in the United States? Does the answer lie in tampon usage patterns or in some other indicator?

Finally, why is this bacterium causing an outbreak of disease at this particular time? "There are three possibilities," says CDC epidemiologist Dr. Bruce Dan. "Women may have changed physiologically—that's unlikely. Tampons may have changed—we know this is true, but don't know what difference it makes. But the most likely change has occurred in the bacterium itself." Researchers are trying to learn how and why Staphylococcus aureus—a fairly common bug, after all—transmuted into a killer with a preference for young, menstruating women.

Tampon companies are also conducting or sponsoring TSS research. Procter & Gamble assigned one of the company's senior scientific directors the task of overseeing a TSS program. Other tampon makers are cooperating with the FDA and CDC in their attempts to understand and treat TSS.

So far, the treatment for TSS victims has hardly changed since the early days. In other words, patients are given large amounts of fluid to offset the dehydrating effects of fever and shock, and they're monitored very closely (sometimes in intensive care units of hospitals) to make sure their vital systems are recovering. Antibiotic therapy has had only limited success; S. aureus is resistant to penicillin and penicillin-like drugs, and beta-lactamase-resistant antibiotics seem to be effective only in reducing or preventing recurrences of the disease, not in curing the original outbreak. This is because the antibiotics kill only the bacteria and do not neutralize the toxin which has already been produced.

But there are some encouraging signs. Microbiologist Patrick Schlievert claims he's isolated a specific S. aureus toxin that produces TSS symptoms in laboratory animals. Since it's the toxin, not the bacterium as a whole, that's responsible for the disease, it may not be long before an antitoxin is developed. Schlievert thinks the answer to the antitoxin dilemma may lie in pooled gamma globulin—an antibody extracted from the blood serum of healthy people. He also hopes it won't be long before women can be screened to find out whether they stand a higher than average chance of getting TSS.

Meanwhile, public education about TSS must play a major role in limiting the disease. In areas where consumers and doctors are well informed about what to do if TSS strikes, cases have been noticeably milder than in areas where surveillance is halfhearted and public education is sparse.

Questions and Answers About TSS

Q. *When is a woman most likely to get TSS?*
A. In studies conducted by the state of Wisconsin and by the federal Centers for Disease Control, 95 percent of the TSS cases occurred in menstruating women. Most of these women first experienced symptoms of the disease on the third or fourth day after menstruation began, but a few women came down with TSS as late as a week after their periods started.

Q. *What are the symptoms of TSS?*
A. The strict case definition of TSS includes a fever of at least 102 degrees, low blood pressure, sunburn-like rash

and subsequent peeling, and the involvement of at least three organ systems (kidney, liver, heart, etc.). All of these symptoms must be documented in medical records. Nausea and vomiting may occur; onset is almost always sudden, like food poisoning. Remember, though, that there have been fatal cases of TSS in which peeling never had a chance to occur, and there have been severe cases in which women never managed to see a doctor. These cases are considered only "probable" by the CDC.

Q. *If I use tampons during only part of my period, will I be less likely to get TSS?*

A. Limited use is the recommendation of the FDA and CDC. But Linda Imboden, the California woman who developed gangrene as a result of a very severe case of TSS, had used tampons for only two days of the menstrual period during which she became ill; she used mini-pads on the other days. Apparently, if you're susceptible to the toxin that causes TSS, it doesn't take much encouragement for the toxin to affect you.

Q. *I'm 36, and my doctor told me I was too old to get TSS. Is this true?*

A. No—although statistically speaking you're at less risk. TSS has been diagnosed in menstruating women as young as 12 and as old as 52. Children, nonmenstruating women and men have also gotten the disease. However, the *majority* of cases have involved women between the ages of 12 and 25—and a third of the cases occur in women between 15 and 19. Women under 30 are three times more likely to get TSS as women over 30—but no one is sure why. Dr. James Todd, the Colorado pediatrician who first identified TSS, speculates that "the older the patient, the more likely she has previously encountered the toxin and developed immunity."

Q. *Isn't Rely the only tampon brand associated with TSS?*

A. No. All tampon brands have been linked with TSS. However, a Centers for Disease Control study conducted in the summer of 1980[5] found that Rely had been used by almost three quarters of the group of women studied, as opposed to only about a fourth of a control group. Shortly after, Rely's makers recalled the brand.

But TSS cases continue to occur in women who use other tampon brands. Minnesota state epidemiologist Dr. Michael Osterholm said that since the Rely recall, the greatest number of TSS cases seemed to be associated with the most absorbent tampon on the market, the second greatest number of cases with the second most absorbent tampon, and so on. Disclosure of brand information is being withheld until publication of the study.

Q. *I've been having some diarrhea on the first couple days of my period. Does this mean I have TSS?*

A. Maybe. Some women seem to have a *normal* pattern of slight constipation just before their periods and slight diarrhea when their flow begins. This is *not* TSS. Neither is dysmenorrhea—the medical term for painful menstruation.

TSS is characterized by diarrhea, sudden fever, nausea and vomiting and—sometimes—rash, shock, and peeling of skin on hands and feet. Very often these symptoms appear to be gastrointestinal flu symptoms. The important thing to keep in mind is that TSS hits very quickly, sometimes within an hour or so, making it more like food poisoning than like flu.

If you suddenly experience diarrhea, fever or nausea during your period and are wearing a tampon, *take it out immediately*. This simple measure may make the difference between a severe and a mild case of TSS. Then call a doctor.

Q. *Can TSS be transmitted to family members or sexual partners?*

A. Possibly. There have been no cases reported of sexual transmission of the disease. However, two sisters in

Minnesota were diagnosed as having TSS, and there have been other reports of sisters getting different versions of the disease. Yet there are plenty of cases in which only one person in a household became ill. It's an area that needs more research.

Q. *Is it possible to get TSS more than once?*

A. Yes. Nearly a third of all women who get the disease have recurring episodes. Certain antibiotic medicines seem to reduce or eliminate these recurrences. However, the only women who've received these antibiotics have been those with cases severe enough to land them in a hospital.

Q. *I think I may have had TSS back in 1975. What should I do about it now?*

A. Many TSS cases currently being reported actually occurred in the past, but are only now being correctly diagnosed. To report your illness (and become a TSS statistic), you must have been under a doctor's care and have medical records documenting blood pressure, temperature and other indicators. If you did see a doctor, contact him or her and explain that you would like to report to your local (city or county) health department. The local agency will, in turn, report to the federal Centers for Disease Control.

If you still occasionally experience symptoms, *do not use tampons.* See a doctor—you may have to see more than one doctor before you find one who is both informed and sympathetic—and ask to have a vaginal culture for Staphylococcus aureus. Meanwhile, give the doctor a detailed description of your illness; any documentation you might have, such as a journal, will be helpful.

Finally, you should be aware that people who have had TSS—especially those who have had severe cases—may later develop cardiovascular problems. This is because the disease causes aneurysms—dilations of the blood vessels. If you've had TSS, watch your diet and exercise as if you were a heart patient, and have regular cardiovascular checkups.

Q. *If I stop using tampons altogether, does that mean I can't get TSS?*

A. Not necessarily. TSS isn't caused by tampons—it's caused by a toxin produced by Staphylococcus aureus, a bacterium. TSS has been diagnosed in young children, in men, in women just after the delivery of a child, and in post-menopausal women. In the nonmenstrual cases, there's generally a localized infection—a skin abscess, for example—that provides a breeding ground for Staphylococcus and its toxins. In menstruating women, the entire vagina is the site of infection. And once you've experienced a severe case of TSS, you may have recurrences even after you stop wearing tampons.

Q. *Is there a test that will tell me whether I might get TSS?*

A. No. It *is* possible to test for the presence of Staphylococcus aureus in the vagina. However, according to Dr. Richard Sweet, chief of the obstetrics and gynecology infectious disease unit at San Francisco General Hospital, "Just because you don't have Staph. today doesn't mean you won't have it tomorrow." Moreover, although positive cultures of Staphylococcus aureus have been taken from women who've had TSS, not every woman who carries the bacterium will necessarily get TSS. According to Dr. James Todd, "not all Staphylococcus aureus can produce the toxin that causes TSS." One of the puzzles about TSS is why—and how—some people develop a defense mechanism against the toxin.

Q. *Everyone says that TSS is a very rare disease. If that's so, hasn't it been overdramatized in the media?*

A. It depends on how you look at it. TSS *is* relatively rare—it strikes only between three and fifteen women out of 100,000 each year. Statistically speaking, you're more likely to die in an auto accident than develop TSS.

However, TSS is less rare for women in some age groups than for others. Women between the ages of 15 and 19 who use tampons seem to be five times more likely to develop symptoms than women ages 40 to 49.

A disease that strikes healthy teenage women is a baffling phenomenon, not only to doctors and researchers but to the press as well. And that's not necessarily a bad thing. Yes, some people are alarmed by stories of an "epidemic." But women who had TSS before it was well publicized knew a much more serious kind of alarm—the kind that results when doctors don't know how to diagnose, or treat, their illness. Steady news coverage of TSS, combined with good doctor education about the disease, has been effective in some areas in reducing the number of severe, life-threatening cases of TSS.

And even though the role tampons play in the development of TSS is still unclear, publicity about tampons' association with TSS hasn't been merely sensational. It's made women more aware that they knew little about what had been a generally accepted, widely used product. It's drawn public attention to the question of how tampons are tested, manufactured, marketed and regulated. And it has stimulated the medical community to continue looking into the relationship between tampons and illness and injury.

NOTES

1. James Todd, Mark Fishaut, Frank Kapral and Thomas Welch, "Toxic-Shock Syndrome Associated with Phage-Group-I Staphylococci," *The Lancet* 2:1116 November 25, 1978.

2. Jeffrey P. Davis, P. Joan Chesney, Philip J. Wand, Martin LaVenture and the Investigation and Laboratory Team, "Toxic-Shock Syndrome: Epidemiologic Features, Recurrence, Risk Factors, and Prevention," *The New England Journal of Medicine* 303:1429, December 18, 1980. The same issue contains reports by a Centers for Disease Control research team ("Toxic-Shock Syndrome in Menstruating Women: Association with Tampon Use and Staphylococcus Aureus and Clinical Features in 52 Cases," page 1436) and an editorial, "Staphylococcal Infection in the Toxic-Shock Syndrome," (page 1473).

3. "Follow Up on Toxic-Shock Syndrome," *Morbidity and Mortality Weekly Report.* 29:441, September 19, 1980.

4. "Toxic-Shock Syndrome—United States, 1970–1980," *Morbidity and Mortality Weekly Report*, 30:25 Centers for Disease Control, Atlanta, Ga., January 30, 1981.

5. "Follow Up on Toxic-Shock Syndrome," *Morbidity and Mortality Weekly Report.* 29:441, September 19, 1980.

6. Arlan F. Fuller Jr., Morton N. Swartz, John S. Wolfson, and Ronnie Salzman, "Correspondence," *New England Journal of Medicine* 303:881, October 9, 1980.

CHAPTER 5

Who's the Watchdog?

In Japan, tampons and sanitary napkins must conform to standards set by the Japanese Ministry of Health and Welfare. Tampons must be free of dyes, fluorescence, acids and alkalis. They must absorb a certain minimum amount of fluid in a specified length of time, and they must leave no more than 1 percent residue after being boiled and filtered. Tampons and their withdrawal cords must be strong enough to withstand being pulled at a certain amount of tension. Tampons that have more than a minimum number of bacteria may be rejected. So may tampons that contain "foreign matter."

But in the United States, there are no government-set standards for tampons. In fact, throughout the history of the commercial tampon industry the government's policy toward tampons has been one of benign neglect. When the 1938 Food, Drug and Cosmetic Act was written, tampons were considered "cosmetics," perhaps the lowest priority item on the Food and Drug Administration's agenda. The agency's only authority over cosmetics was to make sure they weren't adulterated or misbranded; it could conduct occasional inspections of tampon production plants to make sure that "good manufacturing practices" were being followed, but it couldn't oversee tests or require contents labeling. In 1968, the FDA reclassified tampons as "devices"—but the change was only semantic. It wasn't until 1980 that the FDA decided that tampons were a "Class II" medical device subject to "performance standards." Yet actual performance standards still haven't been written.

How did tampons manage to escape government scrutiny in the United States for so many decades? The fact that they are used exclusively by women—and menstruating women in particular—may have had something to do with it. Menstruation is still a taboo subject for a large number of people, bureaucrats among them, and sometimes that taboo gets translated as repugnance: Who could possibly imagine testing—handling, smelling—a used tampon?

But inertia played at least an equal role. Since commercial tampons were on the market five years before the Food, Drug and Cosmetic Act of 1938 without much hue and cry about their health risks, it probably seemed reasonable to the FDA to allow manufacturers to regulate themselves.

Which is pretty much what happened in the late thirties and forties. Tampon companies sponsored medical research, and the results got published in medical journals. Coincidentally or not, the results in those early years generally supported the tampon makers' claims of safety and effectiveness. (See Chapter 3 for more on the history of tampons.) If tampon companies were already doing a good job, the FDA may have reasoned, why meddle?

What has happened since the 1940s, though, is that tampons went from being a discretionary item—something you had to go out of your way to buy—used by a small minority (about 5 percent of menstrual-age women around 1940) to being a virtual necessity for nearly three quarters of all American women of menstrual age. As more women used tampons, it became more likely that eventually a few (or more) of them would develop problems as a result. And when tampon companies began reformulating their tampons in the early seventies, using more absorbent fibers, adding fragrance or changing the composition of the inserter, the likelihood of problems increased.

From 1938 to 1968, the FDA classified tampons as cosmetics—defined by the federal Food, Drug and Cosmetic Act of 1938 as anything "intended to be rubbed, poured, sprinkled, or sprayed on, introduced into, or otherwise applied to the human body or any part thereof for cleansing, beautifying, promoting attractiveness, or altering the appearance." (Apparently the government thought tampons "cleansed.") The government could seize cosmetics if they were "filthy" or "putrid," or it could ban them if they contained ingredients found to be harmful (as it did in 1972 with over-the-counter skin cleansers containing hexachlorophene), but it couldn't inspect manufacturing sites on a regular basis and it couldn't demand to see information the manufacturer thought was "proprietary"—a trade secret. And it couldn't require manufacturers to tell consumers what ingredients were in their products.

So tampons were considered essentially outside federal regulation until the FDA transformed them into "devices." A device is defined by the FDA as "an instrument, apparatus, implement, machine, contrivance, implant, in vitro reagent or other similar or related article . . . which is . . . intended for use in the diagnosis of disease or other conditions, or in the cure, mitigation, treatment, or prevention of disease in man or other animals, or to affect the structure or any function of the body of man or other animals" without using chemical or metabolic means. (In this case the FDA decided tampons "affected a function of the body" of "man.") But reclassification didn't mean more intense scrutiny of tampons' manufacture, partly because the FDA hadn't yet determined just how significant a device tampons were. It took the Medical Device Amendments of 1976 to even permit the prioritizing process to begin.

In Congressional hearings in 1973 and 1975, while the

Medical Device Amendments were being written, consumer advocates in the Washington, D.C.–based Health Research Group testified that there should be mandatory testing of all "implantable" devices before they went on sale. The Health Research Group felt that tampons were implantable devices. But Congress, under industry pressure, eventually approved a watered-down amendment that defined "implantable" devices as only those that remain in contact with body tissues for at least 30 days—which tampons, under normal use, do not.

The 1976 amendments gave the FDA authority to ask for the contents and formulas of tampons without a "compelling reason" and they required the FDA's Bureau of Medical Devices to classify each medical device into one of three categories. Class I, which includes such devices as tongue depressors, requires only "general controls" of the manufacturing process. Class II, which includes hard contact lenses and hearing aids, requires performance standards. Class III, which includes heart pacemakers and IUDs, requires pre-market testing. Because of the enormity of the classifying task, it wasn't until April 3, 1979, that the classifications of obstetrical and gynecological devices were published in the *Federal Register*, the first step toward becoming regulation. (Some devices still haven't been classified, either because they're so new or because the FDA hasn't figured out how to pigeonhole them.) Tampons were separated into "scented" and "unscented" categories, but both kinds of tampons were designated Class II, as were scented menstrual pads. Unscented pads were put in Class I.

The regulation went into effect on February 26, 1980. However, the FDA still couldn't—and can't—require tampon manufacturers to inform consumers about contents. And although the 1979 regulations referred to the need for a biocompatibility standard for tampons "to prevent an adverse tissue reaction" and material standards "to control material absorbency and the wet strength of the removal string," those standards still haven't been devised, two years later.

Ironically, in 1977 the FDA also changed its policy toward cosmetics. That was the year cosmetics manufacturers had to begin listing for consumers all the ingredients of their products. If tampons had remained a cosmetic in the eyes of the FDA, we would today have the contents labeling on tampon packages that many women are now asking for.

The FDA and the Tampon Makers

There's a loophole in the Medical Device Amendments as they apply to tampons. Lawyers call it a "grandfather clause," and this is how it reads:

A device that is first offered for commercial distribution after May 28, 1976, and that is substantially equivalent to a device classified under this scheme, is classified in the same class as the device to which it is substantially equivalent.

What this means is that a new tampon is just like an old tampon as long as it's "substantially equivalent." It means that when Procter & Gamble introduced Rely on a national basis in 1980, it could describe its product in package inserts as "a revolutionary new kind of tampon . . . everything about Rely is different"—and the FDA would still consider Rely to be "substantially equivalent" to tampons on the market before 1976 and thus not subject to government-reviewed pre-market tests. A tampon is a tampon is a tampon, seemed to be the FDA's way of viewing it, even though in this case a tampon was something very unfamiliar indeed.

And the FDA knew that Rely was different. At least four times between December 1976 and July 1980, Procter & Gamble submitted product modification notices to the FDA.

Each time the company claimed that the modification would leave Rely "basically unchanged." Yet the proposed modifications included changes in the absorbent materials in the tampon and the addition of perfume. (Perfumed Rely never made it onto the shelf, though.)

Other tampon makers submitted their own product modification notices during this period too—a voluntary procedure—and in no case did the FDA find that any of these modifications substantially altered the tampon. As Robert Leflar, staff attorney of the Health Research Group, pointed out in a hearing of the FDA's Ob-Gyn Device Advisory Panel, "In the absence of safety testing of these new products, reviewed by this panel and by FDA, it is difficult or impossible to tell whether these product modifications were innocent, or whether they created the conditions for the recent rapid increase in the incidence of toxic shock disease."

If the FDA can't prescribe safety tests for tampons, and if it hasn't yet gotten around to writing performance standards, what *can* it do to regulate tampon manufacturers? It does have the power to recall a dangerous tampon, but it's never done so. Procter & Gamble voluntarily recalled Rely in September 1980, after 71 percent of the 50 TSS cases in a Centers for Disease Control study were linked to Rely use.

The FDA's primary function in regulating tampons is to inspect production and administrative facilities at least once every two years, more often if it seems warranted. But it wasn't until 1976 that procedures for such inspections were established. Before that date, FDA inspectors visited tampon companies only in response to consumer or physician complaints. And, understandably, tampon makers weren't always delighted to see an inspector turn up.

For example, according to a document obtained from the FDA's New Orleans district office under the Freedom of Information Act, an inspector tried to visit Kimberly-Clark Corporation's Conway, Arkansas, plant on July 4, 1974, apparently to follow up on consumer complaints about vaginal lacerations from Kotex tampons. Kimberly-Clark refused to allow the inspector in the plant on grounds that the company's tampons were not subject to the Food, Drug and Cosmetics Act of 1938. After getting a court-ordered inspection warrant, the FDA tried again, on August 23, 1974. This time, when the inspector arrived he found the tampon production line had been shut down. He was "unable to confirm any actual practices regarding quality standards."

According to the same document, there were more complaints about lacerations in 1979, and in early 1980 the FDA once again inspected the Conway plant. The report of this inspection reveals that Kimberly-Clark officials refused to allow the inspector to take photographs of the production area. They also refused to supply the inspector with copies of master drawings of certain production lines or with a copy of the company's recall procedures. The inspector discovered many deficiencies in the plant's accounting and quality control procedures, and he noticed lint, machine oil and grease on machinery that carried tampons. The result was a document citing Kimberly-Clark for multiple deviations from the Code of Good Manufacturing Practices for medical device manufacturers.

However, by September 1980, when the same inspector returned to the plant, the company officials were cooperative and plant procedures had been cleaned up remarkably. No objectionable conditions were cited this time. However, the inspector did note in his report that in the company's files there were recent consumer complaints about vaginal ulcers, lacerations and other problems.

At least in this instance, the FDA seems to have done an effective job of pressuring a tampon maker to conform to hygienic and aboveboard manufacturing procedures. Of course, by September 1980 the specter of toxic shock syndrome was worrying tampon makers as much as it was worrying tampon users, and it may have been a strong incentive for this particular manufacturer to improve its production facilities.

(By the way, the versions of the inspection documents

that the FDA makes available to private citizens under the Freedom of Information Act are heavily censored. References to the actual number of consumer complaints are deleted. So are huge sections of the information about raw materials, as in "The [deleted] is received from [deleted] and is simply identified as [deleted] number [deleted]." All of this information is considered by manufacturers to be proprietary and confidential, and the FDA respects the manufacturers' wish to keep it from the public.)

Apart from inspecting facilities, the FDA stayed out of tampon makers' business until October 1980, when the agency proposed a TSS warning label to be used on all tampon packages. The proposal remains stymied for a number of reasons. For one thing, some tampon manufacturers voluntarily added warning labels to their packages. (However, no two companies used the same wording, a fact which caused confusion among consumers.) Second, Tampax Incorporated (one of the companies that *did* add a warning, but as an insert) objected that there isn't enough evidence linking TSS to tampon brands other than Rely to prove a need for mandatory package labels. Third, some conflicting reports about TSS came out in January 1980: The Centers for Disease Control said that TSS incidence was dropping, and that Rely's recall had eased the problem; meanwhile, the coordinators of a study in Minnesota, Wisconsin and Iowa—three states with superior TSS surveillance systems—claimed just the opposite, that Rely's withdrawal had had no effect on TSS rates, and that all tampon brands were implicated.

Finally, the political climate in early 1981 was not favorable to new regulations of any kind. Before the TSS warning label could be mandated, the CDC's January findings had to be reviewed and the language of the warning approved not only by the FDA Commissioner but also by the Secretary of Health and Human Services—an unusual procedure for an FDA document, and one that probably wouldn't have been taken under the Carter administration. In any event, the delay in getting TSS warning labels may not be as long as it seems. A warning label on liquid protein supplements took more than three years to move from proposal to approval. "Considering how 'quickly' we generally move," said one FDA official in the agency's Rockville, Maryland, headquarters, "this really hasn't been so bad."

The FDA and the Consumer

With the participation of 24 health care associations (which represent about 250,000 health professionals), the FDA has since 1976 kept a computer file called the Device Experience Network (DEN) for consumer complaints about medical devices. Most of the DEN reports come from doctors, but consumers can also file complaints directly into the network or through any FDA district office (see Appendix for locations). Tampon makers, however, like other device manufacturers, are under no obligation to submit the consumer complaints they receive to the DEN.

Recently there's been a dramatic increase in the number of reports in the tampon DEN—from 59 in August 1980 to 590 in February 1981. Many reports cite more than one case of injury or illness.

Although much of the increase is due to reporting of TSS cases, the DEN covers a wide variety of tampon-related problems. One doctor, for example, wrote of seeing 27 patients in two months with "painful vaginal ulcers" that the doctor attributed to deodorant tampons. A woman reported that her physician had told her of four patients besides herself who had developed "abrasive ulcers" from the use of Tampax Slender Regulars. Another doctor treated two cases of injury to the vagina from the use of Kotex Stick tampons. Still another physician reported "two extensive— needing medical intervention—lineal breaks in the sensitive mucosa of the vaginal wall" from the use of Playtex tampons with plastic inserters. (Another doctor expressed the opinion that plastic inserters "should be taken off the market.")

Many women have complained that various superabsorbent tampons—and especially Rely—are difficult or even "impossible" to remove. One wrote that it felt like her "entire reproductive system" was being pulled out when she tried to remove a Rely tampon. Others noted that some tampons left fibers in the vagina, where they caused infections.

The FDA advises caution in interpreting their DEN reports. "The majority of DEN reports are voluntarily submitted by various health care professionals," states a cover letter to the copy of the DEN obtained through the Freedom of Information Act. Furthermore, "DEN data is not statistically based" and "the appearance of a report on a DEN printout does not confirm the validity of the complaint or imply that corrective action is associated with the event." The FDA *may* follow up complaints with investigations of tampon manufacturers. But because information about consumer complaints received directly by tampon manufacturers is deleted in copies of FDA inspection reports released to the public, it's impossible to tell which complaints resulted in inspections or other FDA action.

In September 1980, the FDA began taking a more active role in soliciting the comments of tampon users. Reacting to the publicity about toxic shock syndrome, the Bureau of Medical Devices requested that FDA regional and district offices follow up on all complaints of injury—including ulcerations and lacerations—or death associated with tampon use. A seven-page report form used by the San Francisco district office asked for medical and menstrual history, "hygiene" habits and history of recent sexual contacts. The information was gathered by the district offices and sent to the Bureau of Medical Devices in Rockville, where it's available for review by the bureau's ob-gyn advisory panel.

The FDA and the Sea Sponge

It took the FDA almost 40 years to decide to regulate tampons as medical devices. It took the agency only a matter of weeks to decide to do the same with an increasingly popular alternative to tampons—sea sponges.

Sea sponges, harvested from the world's warm oceans, dried and cut into egg-shaped pieces, have been used as tampons for years (possibly centuries) by a small number of women. (See Chapter 7 for more on the history and suggested use of menstrual sponges.) In the mid-1970s they gained new advocates among "back-to-the-earth" women and women in the feminist and health movements who were beginning to suspect that commercial tampons were not as safe as they were claimed to be. A modest but growing sponge distribution industry sprouted, made up mostly of women who weren't pleased with what they saw as a male-dominated, profit-hungry tampon industry.

Sponges and their distributors might never have concerned the FDA if it weren't for two connected events. The first was the disclosure in the fall of 1980 that two women who'd contracted toxic shock syndrome had been using sponges, one of them exclusively. The second event was inspired by the first. The head of the University of Iowa's hygienic laboratory, Dr. William Hausler Jr., decided to find some sponges and test them for contaminants. He sent a female associate to the Emma Goldman Clinic for Women in Iowa City to purchase a dozen of the sponges on sale there. The sponges were bleached, of the Mediterranean silk variety, and Hausler tested them just as they came out of their plastic packages—without rinsing or boiling them. No one at the Emma Goldman Clinic was told that the sponges were being investigated.

Hausler had access not only to gas chromatography-mass

spectroscopy equipment, but also to a computer that could give him a printout of specific contaminants found in the sponges. He also cultured the sponges for bacteria.

His findings included hydrocarbons (possibly from oil spills in the ocean), nicotine and other substances found in cigarette smoke, "entrapped" sand particles and a raft of common bacteria. Staphylococcus aureus, the bacterium associated with toxic shock syndrome, was *not* among them.

Proceeding on the assumption that a sponge functioned exactly like a commercial tampon—it was a foreign object in the vagina, it was "mechanically" introduced and removed, and it absorbed vaginal fluids—Hausler published a report in October 1980, headlined "Toxic Shock Syndrome: The Sea Sponge is not a Recommended Substitute for Tampons."[1] However, the paper dealt less with sea sponges' association with TSS (which could only be guessed at) than with the substances actually found in the sponges. From his limited study of 12 sponges of one species and from one origin, Hausler concluded that it would be "judicious" to avoid using *any* sponge for menstrual purposes. He seemed particularly disturbed that "there are no controls on the levels of pollutants occurring in a 'natural' product."

The press release announcing the report was quickly copied by dozens of newspapers around the country, and the Emma Goldman Clinic decided to stop selling sponges. Under some FDA pressure, the clinic also undertook a complete recall of every sponge it had ever sold. And the FDA announced in December that it would be investigating all firms marketing sponges "to determine if regulatory action is needed." In the meantime, anyone who wished to legally sell menstrual sponges would have to get FDA approval to sell them as "investigational devices." Sponges sold simply for "personal care," without instructions for menstrual use, were *not* medical devices and thus not under the jurisdiction of the FDA.

As the FDA saw it, menstrual sponges were relatively new "devices," introduced after the 1976 Medical Device

Amendments. Some sponge distributors and sponge users have disputed this, but haven't been able to prove that menstrual sponges were marketed before 1976.

After the FDA had already begun notifying sponge distributors that they were violating federal regulations, the agency undertook its own bacteriological study of sponges. This time the sample was somewhat larger—25 sponges of the hardhead, silk and wool species. The findings included "macro and micro" contamination—sand and other particles, bacteria and yeast molds. Hydrocarbons weren't tested for. However, the substances that did turn up were sufficient to convince the FDA that, in one press officer's words, "an obstacle of filth" existed.

Some feminists have seen a conspiracy in the FDA's efforts to stop the marketing of sponges for menstrual use. "I don't think the government wants such an economical device to be sold," one women's clinic staff member said bitterly. Said another: "How do we know that tampons don't contain even more awful things?"

That, of course, is a valid question. But it's unreasonable to insist on standards for tampons and no standards for sponges. And the unfortunate fact is that a woman who buys a menstrual sponge has only its packager to rely on for guarantees that the sponge has been cleaned and inspected, and that usage instructions are adequate and safe. Nothing protects her from an unscrupulous distributor who may be out of business by the time she develops a sponge-related medical problem.

Some controls will obviously be needed if the sponge is to be considered a sound alternative to tampons. The first step, though, will be to begin thorough medical studies of sponge users to find out whose claims are more meaningful: the laboratories' or the advocates'.

The Consumer as Watchdog

FDA officials haven't been the only people keeping an eye on the tampon industry. Beginning in the late seventies, a number of women had been trying without success to get tampon manufacturers simply to tell them what was in tampons. Judy Norsigian, administrative coordinator of the Boston Women's Health Book Collective (which published the phenomenally successful health handbook *Our Bodies, Ourselves*), wrote in 1979 to all the major tampon makers. None would supply specifics about tampon contents. All asserted that tampons contained "cellulosic fibers" and did not contain asbestos or "adulterants."

Meanwhile, a Maryland legal secretary/writer/artist, Louisa Watson Peat O'Neil, had been doing some sleuthing on her own. In 1977 she'd been working in a microbiological laboratory when a letter from Tampax Incorporated, crossed her desk. It requested Ames tests—to determine whether a substance could cause cancer—on some raw material being considered for Tampax tampons. "I was very much surprised," O'Neil recalls, "that an Ames test would even be considered. Until then, I had blithely thought, tampons were just little pure balls of cotton. Ha!"

O'Neil placed an ad in the *Washington Post* for research volunteers, and in May 1979 she and the seven women she'd picked formed Woman Health International. Its sole purpose was to study the medical effects of tampons. The WHI librarians read every piece of information on tampons they could find—including patent applications, where they discovered that synthetic fibers had been considered for use. The group also embarked on a letter-writing campaign to make contents labeling of tampons mandatory. Largely through the feminist press, O'Neil urged women to write to the FDA in support of labeling.

In July 1980, more than a year of research paid off in the form of an 11-page report, "Forty-seven Years Later— Are Tampons Really Safe?" (See Chapter 1 Notes) It analyzed the skimpy medical literature on tampons and concluded: "Tampons, introduced as a commercial product in 1933, have never really been sufficiently tested and evaluated for safety."

When the outbreak of toxic shock syndrome made it apparent that O'Neil's suspicions about tampons might be valid—and that the work ahead was more than her small volunteer organization could handle alone—she shared her files with the National Women's Health Network, a Washington, D.C.–based, 6,500 member lobbying group that had been instrumental in (among other things) getting drug companies to insert cancer warnings in packages of estrogen drugs used during menopause. The network took Woman Health International's campaign a step further: It requested that tampons be reclassified as Class III medical devices— devices subject to government-reviewed testing before they were sold, in order to determine whether they were dangerous.

Joining the network women in this demand was the Health Research Group, another Washington-based organization, this one with ties to Ralph Nader's consumer crusade. In September 1980, the Health Research Group called for a Congressional investigation into Rely tampons, charging that Procter & Gamble had reformulated Rely earlier that year and that both the manufacturer and the Food and Drug Administration had been negligent in not informing the Centers for Disease Control. (The investigation never got off the ground because the congressman whose committee would have conducted it was not reelected in 1980, and with him went the impetus for a probe.)

Then, in October, Woman Health International, the Health Research Group and the National Women's Health Network each sent a representative to a meeting of the FDA's Ob-Gyn Device Advisory Panel. Representatives from International Playtex, Inc., and Procter & Gamble also attended.

The panel saw some startling slides of vaginal ulcerations due to tampon use, and then heard the arguments from the tampon industry and the consumer advocates. Procter & Gamble's vice president of research and development, Geoffrey Place, told the panel that Rely tampons had undergone nine clinical studies in "organizations independent of Procter & Gamble." Nevertheless, Procter & Gamble had recalled Rely in late September, and was now working with the CDC, with state health departments and with university medical centers to study toxic shock syndrome.

Walter Bregman, president of Playtex, described his company's new program to inform the public about TSS. "While there is no evidence that tampons cause TSS," he said, "we recognize the gravity of the concerns that have arisen as a result of the reported association between tampons and TSS." Bregman also defended the Playtex deodorant tampon, asserting that "consumers want it and buy it."

The consumer representatives had different assertions. Judith Beck of Woman Health International endorsed "complete—and we emphasize complete—labeling from fibers to chemicals to warnings to medical contraindications." She also asked that the FDA remove tampons containing superabsorbent fibers or deodorants, and she called for both industry-funded and government-funded research "for a safe, effective, sterile tampon or substitute device."

Robert Leflar, staff attorney for the Health Research Group, urged that tampons be placed into Class III so that the FDA could review all pre-market testing done on them. It was obvious, he said, that tampons "present a potential unreasonable risk of illness or injury." To keep them in Class II would be the "kiss of death," he added: "It would be years or possibly forever before effective standards could be developed."

Elayne Clift of the National Women's Health Network read to the panel a letter from the Coalition for the Medical

Rights of Women, a San Francisco organization and a member of the national network. "Although women have used tampons for many years without harmful side effects," the letter read, "the Coalition believes that the changes in content and manufacturing techniques which have occurred in the last few years have made the tampon a potentially dangerous device for women to use." The coalition called for reclassification, contents labeling and warnings, user information, and physician and consumer education.

Finally, after two days of hearings, the panel voted on recommendations presented by its non-voting consumer member, San Francisco attorney Joan Graff. It took two votes (and the tiebreaking nod of the panel's chairman) to endorse reclassification to Class III. Recommendations about full contents labeling and package warnings, however, passed without debate. But Graff's recommendations that all deodorant tampons, superabsorbent tampons and tampons with plastic inserters be removed from the market were voted down.

It was a qualified victory—even more qualified in light of the fact that the panel's recommendations are not binding on the Food and Drug Administration. In other words, they are recommendations, not mandates. And five months after they were made, no official action had yet been taken on any of them.

How Should Tampons Be Regulated?

By now, even the Food and Drug Administration acknowledges that tampons need to be regulated differently than they have been in the past. Lillian Yin, director of the division of obstetrics and gynecology and radiology in the Bureau of Medical Devices, admitted in early 1981 that "there is a serious problem with [some] tampons as they now exist."

But what's the best way to make sure that the problem—

or problems—are corrected? Here are some of the recommended solutions:

1. BAN ALL TAMPONS.

This extreme—and admittedly unlikely—option got some attention in October 1980, at the height of the toxic shock syndrome publicity. Gloria Allred, a Los Angeles attorney representing a TSS victim in a lawsuit against the makers of o.b. tampons, held a press conference to request that the Federal Trade Commission remove tampons from the marketplace if they did not include package warnings about TSS. To emphasize her point, Allred burned a box of tampons "as a way of warning women that if they do not destroy their tampons, the tampons may destroy them."

But the Federal Trade Commission's jurisdiction over tampons extends only to tampon advertising, not to product bans. At this writing, Allred's request was being handled as a consumer complaint, and the FTC was not at liberty to tell me whether or not investigations of tampon companies were taking place. A product ban, I was told, would be up to the Food and Drug Administration—only if and when it was decided tampons created a serious and uncontrollable hazard to a sizable number of women.

2. RECLASSIFY TAMPONS AS CLASS III MEDICAL DEVICES.

This would mean that the FDA would follow the recommendation of its ob-gyn advisory panel and require government-reviewed pre-market testing for all tampons on a brand-by-brand basis. It would mean that tampons would be considered, in FDA terms, "significant risk devices" not unlike intrauterine devices (IUDs) and heart pacemakers.

This move is being urged by the National Women's Health Network, Woman Health International and the Health Research Group. Tampon manufacturers, on the other hand, feel that it's too radical a step. Like other medical device makers, they protest that more stringent controls result in a lot of paperwork—but not necessarily in better products. The Pharmaceutical Manufacturers Association has estimated the cost to industry of meeting the FDA's medical device rules at more than $300 million a year—a cost that inevitably gets passed along to consumers.

Not everyone at the FDA believes that Class III is the best category for tampons, either. Even putting aside the question of whether a tampon carries the same degree of risk as a pacemaker or IUD, there's the matter of the time lag involved in setting pre-market approval procedures. A tampon maker could skirt the pre-market approval issue entirely by obtaining an investigational device exemption, thus gaining two and a half years to gather data on tampons' safety and effectiveness. In the meantime, the tampon could legally remain on the market. Many people I spoke with believed tampon regulations would be achieved more quickly if tampons remained in Class II and performance standards were written.

3. RECLASSIFY TAMPONS AS A COSMETIC.

It sounds like a step backward—but it isn't quite. Reclassifying tampons as a cosmetic would mean the immediate requirement of contents labeling, which has been a demand of concerned consumers for at least half a decade.

Most tampon makers other than Playtex (which has listed partial contents on its tampon packages since 1975) don't think this is a very good idea—"Consumers don't know what they're looking for," one tampon company vice president told me. And of course, this alternative fails to address the other urgent problem regarding tampons, the lack of government involvement in standards and pre-market testing.

4. LEAVE TAMPONS IN CLASS II, BUT MOVE IMMEDIATELY TO SET PERFORMANCE STANDARDS AND IMPLEMENT CONTENTS LABELING.

Current regulations allow for the setting of biocompatibility and materials standards, to make sure that tampons don't harm the tissues they come in contact with and that their materials are safe and strong. In other words, they provide for a system of evaluating tampons similar to the Japanese government's.

The problem is that the standards have never been set. And until they have been set consumers cannot be protected from production and design practices that may result in plastic inserters that tear the vaginal membranes and in tampons that come apart inside the body, or from potentially harmful ingredients such as fragrance and high-absorbency materials.

In addition, and without moving tampons into Class III, the FDA could require complete contents labeling on packages. Not all consumers may know how to interpret those labels, but they're an important first step toward further consumer education.

5. IMPROVE PUBLIC AND HEALTH COMMUNITY EDUCATION ABOUT TAMPONS.

In an ideal society, the most effective form of regulation would originate in the consumer herself. Well-informed consumers have the power to stop in its tracks any product that's unsafe, uncomfortable or unnecessary.

Unfortunately, most women have had only tampon makers to turn to for advice about tampons. Most doctors, have had only their female patients and staff. The FDA could provide an important service by printing brief fact sheets on tampons that could be available in supermarkets and drugstores and in doctors' offices.

In all probability, none of these recommendations—even an outright ban—would have prevented toxic shock syndrome from happening. It's unlikely that even the most thorough pre-market testing procedures would have turned up a new disease that occurs in only about 15 out of every 100,000 menstrual age women. (One estimate places at 160,000 the number of women who would have had to be screened in order to detect a single case of TSS.)

But better regulation of the tampon industry *could* have heightened public awareness of toxic shock and other potential problems associated with tampons, so that, for example, a woman with a vaginal infection or unusual bleeding would know that she should immediately remove her tampon. The incidence of vaginal ulcers might decrease if consumers and physicians could read on tampon packages about the hazards of prolonged tampon use. And an industry that's watched more closely by government agencies might be less likely to introduce potentially hazardous ingredients to tampons for the sake of an extra percentage of market share.

NOTES

1. William Hausler Jr. "Toxic Shock Syndrome: Sea Sponge is not a Recommended Substitute for Tampons." *Hotline* 16:1 University of Iowa Hygenic Laboratory, Iowa City (November 1980).

CHAPTER 6

Inside the Tampon Industry

Tampons are big business. In 1979, nearly five and a half *billion* tampons were sold in the United States—and countless millions more American tampons were sold in Europe, Africa and Asia. Tampon sales added up to more than $400 million in revenues for the companies that made them.

During the seventies the tampon industry grew by leaps and bounds. Between 1968 and 1978, tampon sales increased 244 percent, while sanitary napkin sales grew by a mere 86 percent. By 1980, it was estimated that 50 million American women used tampons during at least part of their menstrual periods.

Then came toxic shock syndrome, and warnings from doctors and researchers that highly absorbent tampons may present a greater risk of the disease. The tampon industry was thrown into confusion: Procter & Gamble recalled Rely, Kimberly-Clark quietly replaced its superabsorbent tampons with less absorbent varieties on the shelves of supermarkets and drugstores, and all of the major manufacturers struggled to redeem tampons' public image.

Against this tumultuous background Tampax Incorporated—the oldest continuously active tampon maker in the world—made a dramatic move. The company announced an "innovation" that was really a throwback: the revival of the original, all-cotton Tampax tampon that had been phased out in 1978 in favor of a smaller yet more absorbent Slender Regular version. The idea, explained Tampax president E. Russell Sprague, was to offer women the same "pure and simple" product that their mothers had probably introduced them to.

The all-cotton tampon, like "organic" cereals and "natural" cosmetics, probably seems healthier to many women. And it may actually *be* healthier. Rely, the tampon brand associated with 71 percent of TSS cases in a federal Centers for Disease Control study, was made of all synthetic materials; perhaps it followed that the more natural fibers in a tampon, the less risk that tampon would carry. It's a hypothesis that hasn't been proven (or even tested) scientifically—but then again, it hasn't been disproven, either. Certainly the logic of it was attractive to women in the Tampax test markets of Hartford, Connecticut, and Rochester, New York, who bought up "Original Regular" tampons in 1980 without ever seeing advertisements for it.

At a time when other new tampons were depending on such "frills" as fragrance, plastic inserters or heightened absorbency, Tampax seemed to be opting for simplicity and common sense. The decision to bring back Original Regulars was in keeping with Tampax's image as the Old Faithful of the menstrual products industry—solid, steady and committed to providing the public with just one high-quality product.

But how close to the truth is that image? Does being a one-product company really make Tampax superior in the areas of research, testing and quality control? Was Tampax bringing back cotton tampons because the company knew of risks associated with synthetic tampons—risks the rest of us weren't aware of?

Hoping to answer those questions, and curious to see for

myself the inner workings of the tampon industry, I arranged a visit in February 1981 to Tampax manufacturing headquarters in Palmer, Massachusetts.

Inside Tampax

On the Line

Palmer is a small central Massachusetts town of solid-looking two- and three-story frame houses and small businesses. Polish names and Polish-American meeting halls are commonplace in the area. The Tampax plant—a onetime woolen mill—is located in an even smaller offshoot of Palmer, Three Rivers. It's one of five Tampax plants in the United States—the others are in Rutland, Vermont; Claremont, New Hampshire; Auburn, Maine; and Willsboro, New York—and there are factories in Canada, England, France, Ireland and South Africa that produce tampons to be sold in some of the 106 countries where Tampax is marketed. Together they have produced, over the 45 years of Tampax's corporate existence, over 75 billion tampons—more tampons, it's estimated, than all of the other brands combined. In the process, "Tampax" has come to *mean* "tampon" to milllions of women around the world.

My hosts and guides in Palmer were Thomas J. Moore, executive vice president in charge of manufacturing and research (and the chief executive at the Palmer facility); Clayton L. Thomas, M.D., the company's vice president in charge of medical affairs; and Vera J. Milow, vice president of educational affairs. Milow was also visiting—she usually works at Tampax corporate headquarters in Lake Success, New York.

"We don't generally allow outside visitors," Thomas Moore explained to me in a friendly yet cautious manner. He's been with Tampax for 19 years, 14 of them in Palmer. "It's not that we have anything to hide—but information about our machinery and methods is proprietary." That's why I would not be allowed to take photographs in the plant. "We were a little worried," Moore confessed, "that you might have an engineering background and be able to memorize the details of our machinery." I assured him, truthfully, that such was not the case.

As we crossed a hall into the din and hospital-green glare of the factory, Moore explained to me that Tampax is a "converter" of materials. The company buys paper, absorbent fibers, glue, cellophane and all the other components of tampons and their packages from outside suppliers, and puts them together in a unique manner. In contrast, Kimberly-Clark Corporation, which manufactures both sanitary napkins and tampons along with a host of other paper products, owns all the suppliers it needs for production—from forests to pulp mills to printing plants.

I was a little surprised at how few people—I estimated fewer than 50 in all—are at work on this shift, which started at seven a.m. I guess I'd expected rows of assembly-line workers stuffing tampons into cardboard tubes. In fact, the plant is highly automated, and the employees—mostly women, I noticed, and many of them gray-haired—are essentially inspectors who watch the machinery to make sure everything's moving properly. Roving supervisors—also female, but distinguished by their all-white, nurse-style uniforms—check on the inspectors and fill out papers for quality control. Thomas Moore is proud of Tampax's training program, which utilizes teaching machines, video presentations and one-to-one instruction by experienced workers. However, he would not tell me how many people the facility employs ("more than 300," was as specific as he'd get) or how many tampons they produce.

My first stop in the manufacturing process was the production of cardboard tubes that make up the tampon inserter. Three strips of brown paper are wound spirally around a steel cylinder and coated with a mucilage-type glue; a white layer of paper is added as an outer coating. While they're still soft from the glue, the tubes are cut into short lengths and dried on racks. The tampons I followed were Slender Regulars, Tampax's second best-selling absorbency type. (Supers are the number-one choice of Tampax buyers.) When Slender Regulars were introduced in 1978, Moore told me, a questionnaire was inserted into each box. Some of the women who responded complained that the inserter tube—then made of three layers of paper—was "too flimsy." Tampax decided to correct the problem by adding a fourth layer of paper to the tube.

The next stop is at what Moore called "the heart of the operation"—a complex piece of machinery that automatically wraps the absorbent material (in this case, a blend of cotton, rayon and carboxymethylcellulose, which is a form of high-absorbency cotton) in a rayon overwrap, cuts the wadding into short lengths, stitches a waterproofed withdrawal cord onto the wadding and compresses the whole thing into a compact cylinder. One woman keeps an eye on the entire process, making sure a knot in the thread or the cord hasn't caused the machine to automatically shut down, and looking over the finished tampon for defects. A panel of lights and a rear-view mirror inform her of supply shortages or other events that require her attention.

There are plenty of controls built into the machinery: If a tampon happens to go through the line without getting a cord stitched on, it is automatically rejected before it reaches the inspector; a memory device in the machine makes sure that the *right* tampon is rejected. A little later, the tampons are checked yet again to make sure they have a cord before they're individually wrapped in white paper. "We're very concerned that there be a cord on each tampon," Moore explained.

From the stitching and compressing station the tampons are moved along a belt and automatically stuffed into the now-dry cardboard tubes. The same machine cuts shallow grooves into the tubes to provide a better grip for the woman who will eventually use them. An inspector looks at the tampons before they're wrapped in paper, once again checking to see that the cord's there and blemishes aren't. Then each tampon is wrapped in paper, which is printed and given a tear strip as it unfurls off its roll to meet the tampon. The paper wrapping is sealed over the tampon without glue by a machine that presses the paper fibers together.

The wrapped tampons jiggle down twin pulleys designed to reject any tube that doesn't contain a tampon. Another machine detects the presence of metal in a tampon—a rare occurrence, Moore hastened to note, but one that could come to pass if a supplier's shipment of paper or absorbent fiber was "contaminated." If metal turns up in a Tampax tampon, a blue light goes on and the entire manufacturing line automatically shuts down. A management level employee must start the system again using a key.

The tampons are prepared for packaging by a machine that counts them out—in this case, 40 to a box—stacks them and pushes them into a carton that's been traveling down a parallel line. Automatic controls guarantee the right number of tampons in a box. The only human labor at this station—other than routine inspecting—involves stuffing an informational insert about toxic shock syndrome into each box. The insert advises Tampax users that "TSS is a very rare disease" and that although "tampons do not cause TSS," they have been *associated* with the disease. (In fact, in virtually every case of TSS in menstruating women, a tampon was in place.) It tells women that if they experience a sudden high fever accompanied by vomiting or diarrhea, they should remove the tampon and contact a physician. The insert concludes: "We have been making Tampax tampons for over 40 years and we care!" Although the insert is far from comprehensive, it's one of the more helpful advisories offered by any tampon maker in or on tampon packages. Tampax has been including it in all packages since October 1980.

Finally, the boxes are automatically covered with a cellophane overwrap bearing the brand name and absorbency size. Only boxes of 40s get the overwrap or "discreet" treatment, Moore told me. "That way the woman can remove the wrap and put the box in her bedroom or bathroom, and it won't be obvious that it's tampons." Boxes of 10 tampons, on the other hand, "are more for the woman who wants something to stick in her suitcase or beach bag." Their brand information is printed directly on the cardboard package.

Even after the boxes have been stacked in corrugated cases, they're still not ready to be shipped. A supervisor has to sign all the paperwork that's been accumulating on the line before the tampons can move out of the factory and into trucks for shipping to stores and warehouses.

In the Labs

The bell rang for lunch and the factory, which had been filled with a constant, middle-range machine racket, was suddenly silent. I asked my guides about the purity of the absorbent materials used in Tampax. "They're not sterilized," said Clayton Thomas, "but they don't need to be. The processing they undergo involves great pressure and heat, and it kills just about everything that could grow on the fibers. Not only that, there's never been a case of byssinosis [the 'brown lung' disease that afflicts textile workers] in anyone who works with bleached cotton." (That accounts for the absence of face masks among the factory workers.)

However, Tampax sells tampons in Japan, where government standards require that all tampons be sterilized. So shipments destined for the Japanese market—all produced in Tampax's Auburn, Maine, plant—are sterilized with ethylene oxide gas after they're already in cases. (Ethylene oxide gas was formerly used by various companies to sterilize tampons for the American market. However, that practice was discontinued when it was discovered that the gas left a residue.)

Clayton Thomas is a tall, twinkly, bow-tied man who's been with Tampax for 24 years. His soft Kentucky accent contrasts pleasantly with the flat New England tones of his colleagues. His avocations include sports medicine and ballooning, and he's not above the occasional terrible joke

("My specialty was aerospace medicine—after all, tampons are a form of guided missile").

On our way upstairs to look at the laboratories, we talked about some of the recent bad news about tampons. Thomas had an immediate reply to my questions about tampons and vaginal ulcerations. "Ulcerations can be related to *misuse* of tampons," he said. "In the study, women were wearing tampons continuously for as long as 30 days. Our tampons are designed to be used for menstruation only. I hope to be doing some public-service radio spots to educate women to use the right absorbency and not to use tampons intermenstrually [between periods]."

(In fact, in the study Thomas referred to, published in February 1980 in *Obstetrics and Gynecology*,[1] 10 women who used superabsorbent tampons *during their menstrual flow* developed microulcerations in their vaginal membranes. Chronic tampon use produced even greater incidence of ulceration.)

There are two laboratories in the plant: one for physical inspection and testing of the tampon and tampon package for moisture content, scratched boxes, missing literature and so on; and one for chemical analysis of incoming raw materials, finished products and new products still in development. Once again, most of the employees are women. One was testing some absorbent material to make sure that it contains the amount of carboxymethylcellulose its supplier guaranteed it would. Another was wetting tampons with simulated blood—a mixture of liquid gelatin and red dye—and placing them under weights that simulate the pressure inside the vagina in order to see how much they'll absorb before they leak. Dr. Thomas assured me that the clear red liquid in the tubes has the same viscosity and specific gravity as menstrual fluid. Nevertheless, he admitted that lab tests for absorbency can do no more than provide "kind of a guide." In fact, he said, "The only true, accurate test tube for tampons is the human being." That's why Tampax depends on women volunteers—employees and residents of Palmer—to wear Tampax tampons and turn in the used ones for weighing after they've reached the saturation point.

Thomas had already outlined for me in a letter Tampax's other testing procedures. "When a candidate substance is considered for use in Tampax tampons," he wrote, "we first determine, from the scientific literature, all that is known about its toxic potential. If that investigation indicates the substance is suitable for use, we proceed with certain tests on lower animals, as well as *in vitro* [test tube] studies, the purposes of which are to detect signs of toxic reactions to this material. In addition, we may, depending upon the character of the substance, do specific tests for mutagenicity [tendency to change gene structure] and carcinogenicity [tendency to cause cancer]. If indicated, we have human skin-patch tests done using a rather large number of subjects. Finally, if those tests are all safe, we feel it is in order to proceed with tests in humans." The human panel, however, exists solely to test "efficacy"—that is, does the tampon leak? As for possible side effects of tampon use, Thomas feels that it's long been established that tampons are not only effective but safe.

In the Beginning

Over lunch in the company cafeteria (hamburgers, cheeseburgers, grilled cheese on white bread and fried egg sandwiches, plus an assortment of foods from machines), we talked about Tampax's history. The original patent for Tampax belonged to Dr. Earle Haas, who was born in 1885 and still lives in Denver. (Dr. Haas is also the inventor of the spring used in the arc-spring diaphragm.) Along with some of the founders of Tampax, Dr. Haas was named a decade ago by the *London Sunday Times* as one of the thousand inventors in the 20th Century who had helped make life more comfortable.

Tampax Incorporated was founded by Ellery Mann in 1936 with $300,000; Mann became the company's first president. "He was a great salesman," Thomas Moore recalled. "He'd go out to drugstores around the country and persuade owners to buy Tampax. He was *very* successful. Unfortunately, the drugstore owners weren't as persuasive with their women customers."

Somehow, Tampax managed to survive those discouraging years—as well as the World War II era, when tampon production was cut back in order to produce bandages for the war effort. In 1938, E. Russell Sprague joined Tampax as a junior project engineer and made his way up through management to become president in 1976. He had decided early in his career that he wanted a job in an industry that made a disposable personal care product—and Tampax was his choice. The years revealed just how smart that choice had been. In the 1960s and early 1970s Tampax became one of the most profitable companies ever to sell shares of stock. Back in those days, Tampax was spending only a little over $8 million on worldwide advertising, and was able to claim impressive profits of $29 million on relatively small sales revenues of less than $120 million.[2] Stock market analysts waxed eloquent and prophetic about the company's future, insisting that competitors couldn't make a dent in the market and that Tampax would have the field virtually to itself in the 1980s. As we know, history took a different turn, with first Playtex and then—even more dramatically— Rely gouging out chunks of Tampax's lead. From a 70 percent share of the tampon market in the sixties, Tampax had slipped by mid-1980 to about 42 percent.

But the company was confident in early 1981. It had been able to boost its market share back up to 56 percent. Its all-cotton "Original Regular" tampon had been in test market since mid-1980 with notable success, and "TSS was the final push," said Thomas Moore, for national distribution. The company had taken out an unprecedented half-page advertisement in the *Wall Street Journal* to tell retailers that "in spite of negative publicity, Tampax's consumer sales are up by 15% from the period prior to the recall of Rely."[3] In a "Q and A" interview in the ad, president Sprague asserted that "Tampax tampons have become a way of life for the modern woman," and promised that "Original

Regulars" would be backed by the biggest advertising and promotion budget—$5 million—of any menstrual product in history. According to a *New York Times* report, the message behind the campaign was: "Satisfy your customers as they go back to basics. Tampax introduces cotton absorbent original regular tampons. Women are going back to the name they know they can trust—Tampax—and to cotton, pure and simple."[4]

I asked both Thomas Moore and, in a later telephone interview, Tampax president Sprague, why Tampax had decided to bring back its cotton tampon. Was the company aware of an association between high-absorbency synthetic materials and toxic shock syndrome or other illnesses?

Both men gave me a firm negative reply. And both told me essentially the same thing: Some Tampax customers had simply never liked Slender Regulars. Although Tampax stood staunchly behind its smaller, more-absorbent "regular" product, the company was doing its best to keep every customer—and potential customer—satisfied. Still, it seemed an uncanny coincidence that Tampax had made its decision to bring back Original Regulars at precisely the time when the first report linking ulcerations of the vagina with superabsorbent tampons was published.

In the Classroom

The achievement Tampax is proudest of may be its educational program. Educational affairs vice president Vera Milow, who joined the company in 1952, recalls that this service began just after World War II as a means of teaching store clerks about Tampax's safety and convenience. There was just one problem: Even if clerks were better informed, women consumers still weren't. So a Tampax consultant, Mabel Matthews, developed an outline for teaching "menstrual health." The outline covered a discussion of glands, reproductive organs, the menstrual cycle and general health habits, building up to the history of menstrual products and the advantages of Tampax (as well as instructions for its use, demonstrated on a device called the "Tampax Teaching Model"). The idea was to present menstruation as a normal body function—and Tampax tampons as a safe, modern method of absorbing menstrual flow. With very minor additions and changes, it's the same approach Tampax uses today in its educational presentations.

The menstruation lecture was first brought to nursing students, then to high school and junior high school girls, and most recently to an even younger audience—nine-to-fourteen-year-olds. In the early years, five consultants traveled around the country, staying for as long as two weeks in a community, giving lectures and answering questions. Today there are only three consultants—one in Canada, two in the United States—but Tampax educational materials are in wide circulation: About 10 million copies have been printed of "Accent on You," a booklet aimed at young girls; charts of the reproductive organs and menstrual cycle are available for purchase; and interested consumers can obtain reprints of medical articles on tampons by writing to the company. In addition, Vera Milow goes to at least 20 educational and health conventions a year, offering Tampax informational material—and samples of Tampax tampons—to thousands of teachers, nurses and doctors. The toxic shock syndrome "epidemic" has spurred interest in menstrual education, Milow said. "We've added the Centers for Disease Control's advice about TSS to our presentations."

The latest addition to the Tampax educational program wasn't even in its final edited state during my visit. It's a two-part (one part for girls and boys, one part for girls only), 24-minute film called *Accent on You*, and it is Tampax's first audiovisual teaching aid. I was allowed to see the rough version. Part One presents two self-assured 12-year-olds, Tom and Linda, discussing puberty with an aplomb even an adult would envy. Youthful narrators aside, the program isn't dramatically different from similar "hygiene" films: As usual, male erections are described but not depicted, the clitoris, cervix and hymen go totally unmentioned, and babies and fertilization get ample mention but birth control gets none. Menstrual cramps are downplayed as a matter of poor diet, inadequate exercise and wish-fulfillment. (In this "work print," toxic shock syndrome isn't mentioned, but Tampax officials assured me that the final version would include information about TSS symptoms.) The history of menstrual products is described as an evolution from ignorance and discomfort to enlightenment and freedom. "Until recent years," Linda asserts, "women had no comfortable and convenient way of absorbing the menstrual flow." Now, of course, they have Tampax tampons, which let them "forget all about menstruation." Part Two, narrated by Linda alone, is "girl talk" about menstrual products—with a subtle pitch for Tampax. "Be sure to choose [a tampon]," says Linda, not very grammatically, "that the tubes can be flushed down the toilet." (She must have better plumbing than I do.) She sums up with the usual cheerful advice to see a doctor if you have "any doubts." However, doctors are the first to admit that their knowledge about tampons is sparse.

In General

Back in Thomas Moore's office, we discussed Tampax's past, present and future. My hosts were far from reticent. "We're a unique, one-product company," Moore said.* "We think we've got a tremendous product. We've created an impression on ladies for several generations."

Clayton Thomas agreed. "There's something different about our product," he said modestly. "According to our market share, we should have had 40 percent of the TSS cases. Instead, we had only 5 percent. That's the same percentage as for male and nonmenstruating female cases of toxic shock syndrome."

Nevertheless, both Thomas and Moore acknowledged consumer suspicions about tampons. "Almost half the letters

---

*Actually, Tampax makes plastic tampon containers for sale in the United States, and Tampax's French subsidiary makes a panty liner called "Incognito".

we get are about contents," Moore said. "We always write back and tell consumers what's in our tampons." Such letters say that Tampax tampons are made of "cellulosic materials." Moore continued: "And now we're seriously considering labeling the contents on the box. Although, frankly," he added, "I don't see what help that would be. Most people don't know what they're looking for."

One of the things people have been looking for over the last five years is asbestos, which is known to cause cancer. In 1977, *Well Being*, a "new age" health and nutrition magazine, published an article advising readers not to use tampons because they contained anticoagulants, fiberglass, talc and asbestos. Similar information had already appeared in feminist publications. This time Tampax quickly responded, calling the magazine's claims unfounded, and *Well Being* retracted the article in a 1978 issue. But the damage had already been done: Dozens of other publications, including many women's newsletters, had picked up the information and circulated it. "We continue to be dismayed that people would suspect tampons to contain those harmful ingredients," said Thomas.*

Tampax is currently considering a radical change in one of its hallmark ingredients: the cardboard applicator. Even though Thomas Moore calls the paper applicator "a definite advance—it's convenient, disposable and easy to use," a part-plastic, part-cardboard applicator is being tested "because a lot of women like the plastic." Even if it succeeds, the cardboard applicator would still be available, according to Moore.

The Tampax officials I spoke with express complete willingness to cooperate with the FDA and CDC. They talked with some pride about having passed "three or four" inspections in 1980. According to Clayton Thomas, "We know we're not doing anything different than before the Medical Device Amendments were passed—except a lot of

---

*Also in 1977, the California Occupational Safety and Health Administration tested five tampons and found no evidence of asbestos in any of them.

paperwork." And Tampax officials dismissed the idea of reclassifying tampons into the more strictly supervised category of medical device (Class III), a change that's been proposed by the National Women's Health Network and by the Ralph Nader-affiliated Health Research Group. "There's no proof of need," Thomas Moore insisted.

In summation, Moore said with the confidence that comes from decades of being number one, "The best regulation is the free-enterprise system. Let's face it—if you build a better product, people will beat the proverbial path to your door."

Inside the Other Tampon Makers

Inside Playtex

International Playtex, Inc., is one division of Esmark, Inc., a large and diversified corporation perhaps best known for its Swift & Co. meat-processing business. Playtex itself is diversified, too: Besides being the second-largest tampon manufacturer in the United States, it's the leading maker of women's undergarments ("living" bras and girdles) and also owns Danskin, Inc., makers of tights and leotards.

Playtex entered the tampon business late, by industry standards—not until 1967. It wasn't an auspicious entry. The plastic applicator Playtex used wasn't a hit with women who were used to a completely flushable product. (Plastic tampon inserters are virtually indestructible. I've heard of them washing up on otherwise unspoiled beaches in Tahiti and Hawaii, apparently after being dumped into the ocean from passenger liners.)

What made Playtex a serious contender in the tampon industry was a completely useless innovation: perfumed tampons. Introduced in 1971, "deodorant" tampons followed the successful introduction of other needlessly scented products such as "feminine hygiene sprays," which have been associated with allergic reactions in some women who use them. Playtex managed to straddle the safety issue by telling consumers, on the one hand, that perfumed tampons provided "Deodorant Confidence...during your period that can be reassuring," while on the other hand (and on the same side of the tampon box) cautioning women to "discontinue use if sensitivity or irritation occurs." In interviews, company spokesmen insist that the fragrance in Playtex deodorant tampons has been "extensively" tested at a cost of more than $100,000 per test run.

In any case, 1980 market studies indicated that Playtex was slipping in popularity—and that deodorant tampons in particular had fallen out of favor. In 1978, Playtex captured 35 percent of the American market, but by 1979, that figure had dropped to 31.5 percent—the biggest decline in a single year of any tampon maker. In an attempt to regain some of its former supporters, Playtex reformulated its tampons for greater absorbency in 1980. But that strategy, too, may be backfiring, as information about the association between high-absorbency tampons and vaginal ulcerations—and possibly toxic shock syndrome as well—continues to spread.

In November 1980, Playtex and Johnson & Johnson (makers of o.b. tampons) participated jointly in a public-service advertising campaign to inform consumers about toxic shock syndrome. Playtex also collaborated with Johnson & Johnson (o.b.), Kimberly-Clark (Kotex) and Campana Corporation (Pursettes) to print and disseminate "shelf talkers"—warnings about TSS posted in drugstores and supermarkets where tampons are sold. These warnings repeated the FDA's advice, formulated at the height of the panic about TSS, that women could virtually eliminate their risk of getting TSS by not using tampons. Perhaps to counteract that message, Playtex simultaneously embarked on a massive TV and print media and campaign that featured actress Brenda Vaccaro explaining why Playtex tampons were an "intelligent" choice.

Playtex deserves credit for being the only tampon maker to list at least partial contents of its tampons on the package (rayon polyacrylate fiber, cotton, polysorbate-20, and in the case of deodorant tampons, fragrance). However, Playtex officials would not permit me to visit their manufacturing facilities in Dover, Delaware, and Camarillo, California, or corporate headquarters in Stamford, Connecticut. They would not give me information about testing procedures or names of medical consultants. And they wouldn't tell me whether Playtex tampons were sold in countries other than the United States—that's proprietary sales information, I was told. Yet according to a London newspaper report, Playtex tampons have been introduced in England—where they've met with strong consumer opposition, primarily because of the perfume additive.

Inside Johnson & Johnson

Johnson & Johnson, based in New Brunswick, New Jersey, comprises a wide variety of health-care operations. One division, Ortho Pharmaceutical, manufactures (among other things) diaphragms and spermicides; another, Johnson & Johnson Baby Products Company, makes the familiar shampoo, powder, baby oil and diapers. Other subsidiaries make surgical instruments, bandages, sutures and the basic materials for other J&J products.

Johnson & Johnson Products Inc., another subsidiary, has marketed o.b. tampons in the United States since 1977. o.b. was the first new American tampon without an applicator to be introduced in the last 20 years, and it has captured about 9 percent of the tampon market despite the conventional wisdom that American women are too "fastidious" to insert tampons with their fingers. In fact, o.b. has been a success in Europe since the early 1950s, when it was manufactured by a West German J&J subsidiary. Company literature refers to a woman gynecologist who developed o.b., but company officials will not release her name or address. I was told only that she is "a consultant to one of our European affiliate companies. We respect her professionalism and privacy by not revealing her name, but she is a dynamic and innovative person who is a certified specialist in obstetrics and gynecology."

According to this Johnson & Johnson spokesman, all research and development of o.b. tampons is conducted under the supervision of a staff physician. Raw materials are "patch tested" on the (presumably external) skin of volunteers to see whether they produce irritations or allergic reactions. The raw materials are then put together into tampons, which are worn by J&J employees in in-house tests. When the tampon passes these tests, it's used in clinical tests—again with volunteer subjects—to compare it with competitors' tampons for "effectiveness and acceptability."

Another J&J subsidiary, Personal Products Company (headquartered in Milltown, New Jersey), is test-marketing a scented tampon with a plastic applicator called Assure! Natural Fit Tampons. (It seems that the only way the company is permitted by the broadcast industry code to mention "fit" in television ads is if the word is part of the product name.)[5] Assure! is made of high-absorbency fibers; its advertising slogan is "Assure! Tampons: For a whole new attitude toward your period." In Rochester, New York, one of the test markets, women have indeed been experiencing a "whole new attitude": Several of them have noticed that the tampon falls apart inside the vagina and leaves behind fibers that cause unpleasant odors and infections. When Rochester consumer advocate Judy Braiman-Lipson approached Personal Products with these complaints, "They admitted that they were out for money, that they were fighting for the deodorant tampon market. And they said that of course they wanted their product to be safe, because that meant good business." According to the Rochester *Patriot*, a company spokeswoman told her that "we have a great deal of clinical data that confirms that Assure! presents no safety hazard."[6]

Personal Products also makes Modess, Carefree, Stayfree, and Sure & Natural pads and panty liners. In the past it has manufactured Meds (Modess) and Carefree tampons.

The company produces a booklet, "The Way We Are," that discusses in a fairly sophisticated manner the male and female reproductive systems, conception and pregnancy, venereal disease and—in an afterword—"a message about o.b. tampons and the o.b. method." A Personal Products film, *Naturally . . . A Girl*, is aimed at nine-to-fourteen-year-old girls and their mothers. A toll-free telephone line allows consumers to contact the o.b. Information Center and listen to taped answers to "more than 30 questions about menstruation." (See Appendix for this phone number as well as the names, addresses and telephone numbers of all U.S. tampon manufacturers.)

Inside Kimberly-Clark

The time-honored Kotex brand is the mainstay of Kimberly-Clark's menstrual products line, which includes standard sanitary napkins, beltless New Freedom pads and panty liners, and Kotex Stick and Kotex Security (also known as Kotex tube) tampons.

Kimberly-Clark, headquartered in Neenah, Wisconsin, is a "vertically" organized paper products company, which means it owns everything from forests to mills. It makes a wide range of paper goods, such as Kleenex tissues and paper towels, Kleenex Huggies and Kleenex Super Dry disposable diapers, and papers for tea bags and cigarettes. Tampons are a very small part of the Kimberly-Clark picture—Kotex tampons make up only about 3 percent of the U.S. tampon market—and they've never been as successful as Kotex sanitary napkins.

Kimberly-Clark operates an educational service, the Life Cycle Center, that has provided teaching materials about menstruation since 1922. Booklets with titles like "Very Personally Yours" and "Tell it Like It Is" are available for 10 cents each, and a menstrual physiology chart is free. One of the most famous Kimberly-Clark teaching aids is a Walt Disney-produced cartoon, *The Story of Menstrua-*

tion, that has been shown in schools and youth groups since 1946. In this sanitized, romanticized movie, menstrual fluid is not red but white![7]

Kimberly-Clark seemed unwilling to part with anything but the most sketchy information about its tampons and testing procedures. I was told that "all new components and modified products are thoroughly tested prior to introduction into final product"—but not whether human subjects were used or what kinds of tests were employed. The company "retains recognized experts in the field of obstetrics and gynecology as consultants and medical advisors," I was told, but I could not obtain their names.

Inside Campana

Campana Corporation makes Pursettes tampons, Campana Italian Balm hand lotion, and Ayds diet products. The company is wholly owned by Purex Industries, Inc., which also manufactures Purex bleach, detergent and fabric softener. Purex general offices are located near Los Angeles in Lakewood, California, and Pursettes tampons are made in the old Campana plant in Batavia, Illinois.

Pursettes have been around since the early fifties, when a company called Sanitary Products distributed them on a limited basis. Campana bought Sanitary Products in 1954 and began distributing Pursettes nationally three years later; in 1962, Campana was bought by Purex. This makes Pursettes the second-oldest tampon brand in the United States (Tampax, of course, is the oldest). Ironically, Pursettes is the tampon with the smallest market share—only about 1 percent of American tampon users buy Pursettes.

Despite its modest position in the market, Campana has had an important influence on the tampon industry. It was a Campana consultant, Dr. G. Rapp of Loyola University of Chicago, who invented the "Syngyna," an artificial vagina that (according to a senior Purex official) "duplicates the vaginal site mechanically." To quote again: "By furnishing pressure similar to that to which a tampon is exposed when in use, a more accurate measurement of the actual absorbency can be obtained." The Syngyna is currently used by Pursettes, as well as by most other major tampon makers, to test absorbency.

Purex was obliging in furnishing details of testing procedures used on Pursettes. According to a Purex vice-president, before Campana introduced the brand on a national basis in 1957, the company had the tampons "extensively" tested in animals and, later, in menstruating women. "No adverse effects or vaginal irritations were encountered," I was told. In 1962, when a nonwoven rayon covering was added and the tip lubricant altered slightly, more irritation studies were conducted with female beagles and on the external skin of human subjects. Currently, both raw materials and finished tampons are checked by a staff microbiologist for microbial contamination; finished tampons are also tested for absorbency.

Campana was the only tampon maker that allowed me to see copies of consumer letters—both complimentary and critical. One letter, signed "A satisfied consumer," expressed appreciation that "this personal product" was *not* advertised on television or radio. A less satisfied consumer wrote that a change in the cellophane wrapper on each tampon made using the tampon "like wrestling with a 'child-proof cap.'"

Campana has no educational program, but the instructional leaflet enclosed in each Pursettes box is one of the most comprehensive of its type. The information about toxic shock syndrome, added recently, compares very favorably to what the other tampon companies offer either in package inserts or public service ads. It includes mention of the risk of recurrences of the disease, and it notes, correctly, that TSS has other symptoms besides the "early warning signs" of fever, vomiting and diarrhea. Elsewhere on the leaflet is a caution that "continuous use of tampons during any 24-hour period is not recommended."

The Consumer and the Tampon Industry

As I write this, in spring 1981, the major tampon manufacturers are waging new and aggressive advertising campaigns in the pages of women's magazines. A Playtex ad features actress Brenda Vaccaro defending deodorant tampons as a question of individual "choice" (a word that these days carries inevitable echoes of the abortion controversy). The newest Tampax ad campaign asserts that Tampax tampons contain no "petrochemical sponges" (a reference to the polyester material in Rely), or "potentially irritating deodorant scent" (a frontal attack on Playtex). And there's a three-page ad for o.b. tampons in *Redbook* that assumes a heightened scientific attitude: Instead of fashion models or actresses, there's a woman in a white lab coat peering through a microscope; instead of vague claims about "protection," there's the lofty statement that "Johnson & Johnson maintains constant surveillance of o.b. to insure proper performance."

The fact that tampon companies are courting women so vigorously, and at such great expense, seems to indicate that women are becoming "harder to get," more skeptical. Certainly women are becoming better informed. Also this March, no fewer than three magazines aimed at women— *Cosmopolitan*, *Playgirl*, and *Vogue*—carried articles about menstruation and the menstrual products industry. It's a striking change from the time, not so long ago, when women's magazines maintained an editorial silence about menstrual products, perhaps for fear of offending advertisers.

I think it's a healthy change. It means that many of us are no longer willing to accept that if a big company markets a product it has to be safe. We can no longer be counted on to be too embarrassed to raise pointed questions about menstrual products. We're challenging not only the ways tampons are made and tested, but the ways in which we're persuaded to buy them.

In the months and years to come, we need to keep paying close attention to the messages we hear and read from the tampon industry, for without a doubt, the tampon industry will be listening to the messages it gets from us.

NOTES

1. Eduard G. Friedirich, Jr., and Kenneth A. Siegesmund. "Tampon-Associated Vaginal Ulcerations" *Obstetrics and Gynecology* 55:149 (February 1980).

2. Kathryn M. Welling, "Marketing the Unmentionables," *Savvy*, (June 1980), p. 34.

3. *The Wall Street Journal*, Feb. 20, 1981, p. 6.

4. Philip H. Dougherty, "Tampax 'Original' to Return," *The New York Times*, Feb. 19, 1981, p. D16.

5. Welling, "Marketing the Unmentionables," pp. 33–4.

6. Mickey Revenaugh, "New tampon falls apart, say consumers," *Rochester Patriot*, April 1–12, 1979, p. 5.

7. Janice Delaney, Mary Jane Lipton and Emily Toth, *The Curse*, New York: E.P. Dutton, 1976, p. 95.

CHAPTER 7

Other Ways

A strange thing happened in the last few months of 1980. Up until then, tampon use had been steadily increasing in the United States; in July 1980, about 70 percent of American women were using tampons for at least part of their menstrual periods. But in the fall and winter of 1980, as the news about tampon hazards—especially toxic shock syndrome—was spreading, tampon use abruptly declined. When tampon manufacturers conducted a telephone survey in December, they found that only about 55 percent of American women were still using tampons.

And among those women who did still use tampons, there were growing doubts. "I admit I'm not comfortable with tampons," one woman told me. "I'm worried about the risks—and at times I find tampons *literally* uncomfortable, especially when I'm not flowing heavily. My problem is, I've used tampons ever since I started menstruating. I don't want to give up the convenience. What else can I use?"

Fortunately, there are plenty of options—none completely satisfactory for all women—but the important point is that *women* are now actively seeking to find the best solutions. In fact, one of the promising and exciting consequences of the recent attention given to toxic shock syndrome is that we've all become a lot more aware of just how important alternatives are.

Sanitary napkins

The most readily available alternative to tampons was, in fact, discovered by women. During World War I, some French nurses noticed that the cellulose surgical gauze they were using for bandages made a more efficient menstrual pad than the bird's-eye flannel they'd used (and reused, after washing) during their periods. Not only was it more absorbent with less bulk, it chafed less and was cheap enough to be disposable.

In 1921, the first commercial sanitary napkin was marketed by Cellucotton Products Co. (later Kimberly-Clark, Inc.) under the trade name Kotex, which quickly became a generic term for the product. Six years later, Johnson & Johnson—which had tried, back in 1896, to sell a gauze-covered cotton disposable pad but had been thwarted by advertising taboos—introduced Modess napkins through a subsidiary, Personal Products Co. Other brands surfaced over the years—in 1943 *Consumer Reports* evaluated no fewer than 45—but Kotex and Modess remained by far the dominant names in the industry until 1961, when Scott Paper Company introduced Confidets, a pad with a distinctive "tapered" shape that was packaged together with disposal bags. In 1978, Confidets was the favorite sanitary napkin in a *Consumer Reports* study, but Scott discontinued the brand in mid-1980.

Except for variations such as waterproof linings, or paper construction instead of cotton or cellulose, sanitary napkins didn't change greatly until 1970, when Personal Products introduced its revolutionary Stayfree Mini-Pad. This was a trimmed-down beltless pad that attached to underwear by means of an adhesive strip down the length of the pad. It's been suggested that the mini-pad was an answer to the needs of women who were taking birth control pills and thus had lighter than normal menstrual flows. Whatever the motivation for its development, the new pad and its imitators quickly won acceptance from millions of women who found them comfortable and convenient for the waning days of their periods, for times when they had vaginal discharges, or as a supplement to tampons. Current advertising would have one believe that there's not a day in the month when a mini-pad isn't beneficial!

More recently, the "maxi-pad"—a pad of conventional bulk but with adhesive strips—has joined its smaller counterpart on the shelf. Both mini and maxi versions may contain fragrance, and both have plastic shields to block leaks.

The newest pads are ultrathin because they're made out of the same superabsorbent fibers used in many tampons. Sure & Natural Maxishields, made by Personal Products Company, are nearly as thin as minipads, but they're said to be as absorbent as standard napkins.

Beltless pads offer obvious advantages over old-style pads (which, of course, are still available): there's no belt to show through thin clothing, and there's usually less bulk to contend with. But all external menstrual products pose some risk of chafing, which in hot weather, or when used by women with large thighs, can be extremely annoying. And the beltless pads have a few disadvantages of their own: The very thin ones tend to fold over down the middle, increasing the possibility of stains on underwear, and most of them tend to slip around to some degree. Recent innovations, such as wider or multiple adhesive strips, may solve those problems.

All external pads carry the risk of bacterial infection. Two factors contribute to this risk: Unlike tampons, pads are in contact with the air, whose bacteria find blood and fiber perfect media for growth; and the pad covers the entire perineal region, thus collecting traces of urine and feces along with menstrual blood. In hot climates in particular, yeast and Trichomoniasis organisms may multiply on the warm, moist pads and produce infections. (The same possibility may exist, although probably to a lesser degree, with tampons, because of the "wicking" action of the withdrawal string.)

"Deodorant" pads are more logical than "deodorant" tampons, because odor is an inevitable consequence of napkin use. When the menstrual fluid comes in contact with air, it begins to break down, releasing gases that have a characteristic, and sometimes strong, odor. But perfumes on pads are not necessarily the solution. A dermatologist recently reported seeing a patient whose vaginal lips and anus were inflamed because of a perfumed sanitary napkin.[1] According to his report, the unnamed manufacturer of the napkin subsequently reformulated the perfume, eliminating two of the substances to which the patient was sensitive. But, as this doctor pointed out, "Perfumes are complex mixtures consisting of a few to several hundred individual fragrance components"—any one of which may produce a skin reaction. If you think you may be sensitive to a fragrance in a napkin, switch to an unscented version. And be sure to examine the box carefully: Even a "nondeodorant" product, such as Personal Products' Carefree panty shields, may contain small amounts of perfume. (Carefree is "softly scented," while deodorant Carefree is more heavily scented.) The best advice for menstrual odor is to use unscented pads and change them frequently.

Some of the newest menstrual pads really represent a revival of an old idea. Two women-owned companies in California—Cycles and Scarlet Moon—are currently manufacturing handsown cloth pads and belts on a very small scale. Some are meant to be laundered and reused—just like the rags used by past generations of women. Scarlet even makes a silk pad for the celebration of a girl's first menstruation!

Sponges

Sea sponges have been used as tampons for hundreds—possibly thousands—of years. In the last five or so years, they've been "rediscovered" by women looking for an alternative to fiber tampons. Currently, though, sponges are the subject of an investigation by the Food and Drug Administration, which has become concerned about the marketing of an unregistered and untested "medical device." As a consequence, some women's centers and health food stores that had previously sold menstrual sponges have stopped doing so, or are continuing to sell them but informing women about their potential hazards.

The sponge is an animal, so primitive that for decades it was considered a plant. Sponges are found in warm bodies of water, fresh and salty, throughout the world, although most commercial harvesting takes place in the Mediterranean and Caribbean oceans and the Gulf of Mexico. The species most commonly used for menstrual purposes are the "silk" (caramel-colored—"blonde" if bleached—soft and fine pored, often sold as a cosmetic or art sponge) and "hardhead" (brown, firmer and larger-pored). Occasionally "grass" and "wool" sponges are used as well.

No one knows exactly when sponges first started being used as menstrual tampons in the United States, although I've heard it said that prostitutes used them in the nineteenth century because they didn't interfere with business. But in the early seventies it was young feminist women who were trying sponges. One sponge distributor in the South recalls that in 1975 she was visited by a friend from Tennessee who extolled the convenience of sponges for traveling—you needed only one, which lasted for months. Sally Stevens, who began distributing sponges in 1978, had discovered them in a thrift shop near her tiny community in rural Northern California. "There was a basket full of sponges labeled only 'menstrual sponges,'" she recalls. "Out of curiosity, I bought one and took it home, where it sat for months. I just couldn't put that disgusting-looking thing inside me. It wasn't even *white*!" Once she tried the sponge, though, she never went back to tampons. Soon Stevens was buying bulk sponges from Florida and the West Indies and filling 10 to 15 orders a day. She even bought commercial time on a local radio station.

Sponge distribution is generally a small-time business; the largest distributor I contacted had sold 25,000 sponges in three years. All the distributors I talked to said they inspected their sponges for sand and coral, and some distributors rinsed them as well (one woman rinses them three times). Then they're packaged in plastic or cotton bags; cotton is preferable for storage between periods because it allows air to circulate around the sponge. The cost of sponges varies between $1 and $5 for a package of one or two.

Virtually all distributors include some information about sponge use in their packages. Some advise boiling the sponge before using it, after each menstrual period, or both; some suggest sewing dental floss to the sponge to facilitate removal, while others note that the sponge is easily removed with the fingers. But all emphasize sponges' "naturalness," economy and ecological soundness.

There's nothing particularly difficult or mysterious about using a sponge, although some women confess they had to overcome a certain squeamishness about touching their menstrual blood. A new sponge should be inspected carefully, and any bits of debris still clinging to it should be removed. The optimal size of a sponge varies from woman to woman—some women keep several sponges of different sizes for different times during their periods—but a general guideline is to trim the sponge to the size and shape of a chicken egg. Next, it's rinsed thoroughly or boiled for about twelve minutes (boiling will kill virtually all bacteria and fungi that might be in the sponge, but it also shortens the life of the sponge). After wringing it out until it's almost dry, the woman compresses it with her fingers and inserts it high into the vagina. When it's saturated—usually a little sooner than a tampon would be—she removes it, squeezes out the blood, rinses the sponge in clear water and reinserts it. When no clean water is available, the sponge may be reinserted without rinsing, or it can be placed in a cotton or plastic bag and a fresh sponge reinserted. At the end of the menstrual period, the woman rinses her sponge (or sponges) well, or boils it, and lets it air-dry. A little white vinegar or chlorophyll can be added to the rinse water for a safe, fresh smell. A single sponge, properly cared for, will last several menstrual cycles; some women report they've used the same sponge for a year.

Women who have tried sponges and liked them tend to be wholehearted in their endorsements. One customer wrote to Sally Stevens from an armed services post in Saudi Arabia, "I continue to be surprised and delighted with my sponges after more than a year of use. How great to have these personally molded shapes in my pocket wherever I go." Other women say they like to see how much blood they're losing. "Sponges debunk the myth of genital 'nastiness,'" one woman wrote me. Some women claim that their menstrual cramps became less of a problem when they switched from tampons to sponges. Many women are pleased with sponges' softness, and others like the fact that they're canceling their support for the "feminine hygiene" industry, with its insistence on secrecy and its virtual dominance by men.

Complaints about sponges have been relatively mild: "They leak when I sneeze or laugh hard"; "I never felt really 'protected' with a sponge." Women with vaginal infections should not reuse a sponge, and should either boil or discard a used one. A San Francisco allergist told me of a woman he'd treated several years ago for what turned out to be a reaction to the iodine in the sponge she'd been wearing; she'd developed a rash that went away when she stopped using the sponge. The doctor suggested trying a different species of sponge to see whether it contained less iodine.

In fact, little is known about the chemical contents of sea sponges. Although supporters of sponge use have argued that sponges are safe and ecological, they have done so without laboratory proof for their claims. In August 1979, a group of women from the Cedar Rapids (Iowa) Clinic for Women contacted the University of Iowa Hygienic Laboratory, which does work for the state of Iowa, to find out whether the sponges they were selling could be tested. They were told there wasn't sufficient cause to warrant such testing. But by the following year the situation had changed: Two cases of toxic shock syndrome, one in Minnesota and one in New York, had been linked to sponge use. Intrigued, the Iowa hygienic laboratory's director, Dr. William Hausler Jr., sent a woman colleague to the Emma Goldman Clinic for Women in Iowa City to buy some sponges for testing.

Twelve samples, all bleached sponges of the silk species, were analyzed by means of gas chromatography-mass spectrometry. The findings included sand and coral particles, common bacteria and fungi, and various harmless minerals present in tap water. What drew the most publicity was the finding of traces of hydrocarbons, whose "possible source," said the laboratory report, was an oil spill in the ocean where the sponge had grown.

When I questioned him about the actual health risks of hydrocarbons, Dr. Hausler laughed and declined comment. Dr. Adel Franks of the Emma Goldman Clinic explained that no one really knew what damage hydrocarbons could do to the vaginal mucosa.

There was some evidence of research bias in the sponge study. Dr. Hausler admitted he harbored suspicions about the sponge distributor from the outset. Noting that the sponges were labeled "From the oceans of Iowa," he commented, "We weren't dealing with an organization that was totally up-front. . . . These people were obviously very astute. They knew about restrictions on interstate sale of an unregulated device, so they pretended the sponges weren't brought in from elsewhere." Dr. Franks of the Emma Goldman Clinic had her turn to laugh over that. "It was just a cutesy, innocent slogan," she said. "I believe all the sponges came from the Mediterranean."

Despite the limitations of the study, it was taken seriously by the media, by the FDA and by many women. The Emma Goldman Clinic immediately stopped selling sponges and began, under FDA supervision, to recall sponges it had already sold. (The clinic had been a wholesaler as well as a retailer, selling sponges in bulk to health food stores and other outlets in the Midwest.) The FDA's Bureau of Medical Devices issued a statement to district offices warning that sponges were an unapproved medical device and that distributors would be subject to inspection and registration. In late 1980 and early 1981, FDA inspectors began contacting sponge distributors and wholesalers, telling them that sponges for menstrual use were considered "investigational" devices, and that anyone who wanted to sell them would have to receive an investigational device exemption. To date, no one has done so. However, some women are trying to prove that sponges were sold for menstrual purposes before 1976 when the FDA's Medical Device Amendments were passed. Any device that is "substantially equivalent" to one sold before 1976, can be sold without government-reviewed pre-market testing (see Chapter 5).

Before the Iowa study, the FDA had regarded sponge use as too small a phenomenon to warrant bureaucratic intervention. Some officials did express concern over what they saw as a public health risk: Lillian Yin, director of the FDA's ob-gyn and radiology devices section, told me in early 1980 that she would be upset if one of her children entered a public restroom while a woman was rinsing her sponge. "Suppose a woman has an infection?" she demanded. "What are the chances of it spreading?" But by the next year, this concern was overshadowed by the more basic concern that sponges were not subject to quality control. In their haste to put the lid on sponge distribution, FDA officials often found themselves acting out comic roles. Most had no idea what they were supposed to be inspecting.

"We're pursuing anything that's labeled 'menstrual sponge' or that looks like a menstrual sponge," a San Francisco FDA compliance officer told me. When I asked him what a menstrual sponge looked like, he replied, impatiently, "Well, like a tampon, of course." I explained that a sponge doesn't resemble a tampon at all. "You mean it's not shaped like a tampon?" he said, surprised. "Well, that's news to me."

Some sponge distributors complied with the FDA's new policy and began registering their sponges. Others chose to keep a low profile, stopping advertising but continuing to fill orders, or selling sponges simply as "sponges," for whatever use women might choose to put them to. Many women were suspicious of the FDA's interest in sponges. "I'm disturbed by the way a vague study wasn't questioned," said a woman at the Ithaca (New York) Women's Resource Center. A director of the Berkeley Women's Health Collective said, "We've been selling sponges for five years with no complaints. This recent attention to sponges is weird to me. It seems to be making menstruation a disease again— as though *everything* gives us toxic shock syndrome."

The irony is that only two cases of TSS have been associated with sponge use. There have been more cases of TSS in men, in young children, or in women shortly after childbirth than there have been in sponge users. The problem is that no one has studied sponge users. I spoke with a doctor who had wanted to perform such a study before the FDA became interested in sponges. Now, she said, the investigational device exemption sounded like too big a hurdle.

While sponge distributors were groping toward an alliance that would allow them to afford expensive laboratory studies of their products, a group of four men and one woman in Davis, California, began researching the environments in which sponges grow. Calling themselves the Davis Health Collective, they compiled reports of oil spills and maps of worldwide pollution, and contacted friends in Europe and Asia to collect information about sponge harvesting and use. They hope to substantiate a theory that Chinese women have used sponges for thousands of years with no ill effects, and they want to update the body of sponge research—most of which, according to collective co-founder John O'Donnell, was done more than a century ago.

For women to whom the idea of sponges is appealing, two other uses should be mentioned. One, described in *Hygieia: A Woman's Herbal*,[2] involves sewing sea sponges into a cotton overwrap to make an external menstrual pad. The other, offered as an "emergency" solution in Alicia Bay Laurel's *Living On the Earth*,[3] employs commercial household sponges: Simply cut one into four "sticks," Bay Laurel advises, and insert. This method obviously circumvents the FDA and is even cheaper than sea sponges. However, commercial cellulose sponges are usually dyed, and the effects of dyes on the vaginal membrane are unknown. Perhaps it's best to reserve this method for true "emergencies."

The Diaphragm and the Cervical Cap

Although they're designed for contraceptive, not menstrual use, both the diaphragm and the cervical cap may be used to collect menstrual fluid. In fact, the cervical cap is now considered an "investigational" contraceptive device by the FDA (although it's been used for birth control in England and Europe for decades), and its only approved uses in the United States are collection of menstrual fluid and assistance in artificial insemination.

The diaphragm and the cap are inserted high into the vagina—higher than a tampon or sponge—so that they completely block the opening to the cervix. Of course, no spermicidal jelly or cream should be used during menstruation while the fluid is being collected. The diaphragm employs a spring around its rim; the cap creates suction against the cervix. A doctor or nurse practitioner usually instructs a woman in the proper use of either device. Because conception *is* possible during the menstrual period, the cervical cap may not be a good contraceptive during active menstruation, which can interfere with the cap's suction.

Both diaphragm and cap hold more fluid than a tampon or sponge, but it's advisable to remove and rinse them at least twice a day, even when the flow is light. Regular, extended use of either device *may* pose some risk of cervical abrasion or erosion; not enough studies have been conducted on the use of the cap or diaphragm during menstruation to know how serious the risk is. Self-examination with a plastic speculum, mirror and flashlight is one way to detect changes in the cervix that may indicate the need for medical attention (see Chapter 2 for an explanation).

The Menstrual Cup

The menstrual cup takes the "barrier" principle of diaphragms and cervical caps a step further, adapting it to menstrual purposes. It was sold in the United States from the early 1950s until 1972, when its manufacturer went bankrupt. However, interest in the cup never really died, and in early 1981, plans were being laid to bring the cup back on the market in the very near future.

The origins of the cup closely parallel the origins of the commercial tampon. Shortly after World War II, a ballet dancer, Leona Chalmers, and her physician husband devised a rubber cup that looked like a bell with a ridged open end and a small loop on the closed end. Around the ridge were six tiny holes that prevented a semi-vacuum from being created. The cup was soft enough to be folded for insertion into the vagina, where it lodged between the vaginal muscles at a short distance from the cervix. It had a capacity of one ounce—which meant it could hold as much as half of a woman's entire monthly flow (depending, of course, on the

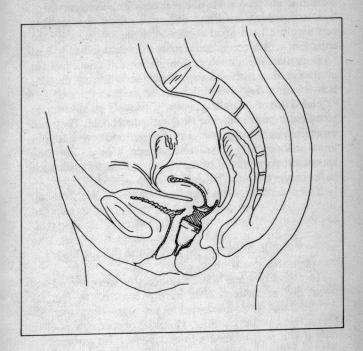

The menstrual cup in place.

woman) before being emptied, rinsed and reinserted. Its creators christened it Tassette—French for "little cup."

It took a while for Tassette to get off the ground; rubber was simply in too short supply after the war. But by the early fifties, when peacetime rubber production had geared up, a facility was established in Stamford, Connecticut, to produce and market the cup. Over the following decade, half a million Tassettes rolled off the assembly lines.

Marketing was another story. Tassette's manufacturers faced three problems. The first was educational: They had a radically new product and needed an intensive informational campaign to familiarize women with it. Yet they lacked the promotional resources of an industry giant such as Tampax or Kimberly-Clark.

The second problem was an "aesthetic" one: The cup was designed to be reused, and some women, accustomed to disposable tampons and napkins, balked at handling their menstrual fluid in such an intimate manner. Women who weren't well instructed about how to use the cup tended to complain that it was messy.

The third problem was economic, for when the educational and aesthetic hurdles were overcome, the fact remained that a single cup lasted for ten years—or longer. No repeat sales, no large profits. This was, of course, a problem only if you were on the profit-making end; for women who tried and liked the cup, its reusability was a definite financial advantage.

Doctors greeted the Tassette with enthusiasm. A New York physician, Rebecca Liswood, cited 12 advantages of the cup over napkins or tampons in a 1959 article.[4] Besides being "clean, safe, sanitary and convenient," the cup was economical and pliable. Virgins, Liswood noted, could use it "without harm."

In 1962, Karl John Karnaky, an early champion of tampons (see Chapter 3), reported on a study of 100 women who used Tassette.[5] He concluded that the cup did not injure the vaginal walls and resulted in far less bacterial contamination than either the sanitary pad or the tampon. So superior was the cup, in fact, that he predicted it would "replace most internal tampons and external pads."

Dr. Eduardo F. Peña of Miami also wrote in 1962 about the advantages of the cup.[6] He studied 125 women, ages 20 to 45, for three months or longer. During their menstrual periods the women emptied the cup twice a day (morning and night), rinsed it and replaced it. At the end of three months, every woman in the study said she found the cup practical, economical, hygienic and easy to insert and remove. In fact, "None would consider using anything but the menstrual cup in the future." Peña concluded that only women with unusually positioned cervixes would have difficulty using the cup. That conclusion was endorsed two years later when a group of University of Michigan doctors reported on 45 women with very heavy menstrual flows (six pads or tampons on the first day) who successfully used Tassette. Twenty-three out of the 45 preferred the cup to their previous menstrual product.[7]

Despite all the professional praise, Tassette was hardly a moneymaker. To remedy the situation, its creators began searching for a cheap, disposable material to replace the long-lasting rubber. They found it in a new, patented, uniquely suitable substance: a "thermoplastic rubber" that softened when it came into contact with body heat. It was not biodegradable, but it could be flushed down a toilet because it was partially water-soluble. When it entered the sewage system, it floated so that skimming equipment employed by large cities' water systems could pick it up along with other floating debris. (The problem of disposal in small towns and rural areas was apparently never addressed.) According to one account, 50,000 of the new thermoplastic cups were flushed into a single sewage system during a one-day test, with no adverse effects.

In 1968, Tassette took its new menstrual cup—renamed Tassaway—to California for test marketing. Over the next three years, the product was introduced into 10 other western states, and plans were laid for national—and even international—distribution. Tassaway was still not a serious challenge to Tampax, but surveys showed that it had garnered a surprising 5 percent of the market. Original forecasts had hoped for 1 percent.

Flushed, as it were, with this victory, the Tassaway people hired a sales manager to promote the cup on a national scale. He took the Tassaway account to J. Walter Thompson, one of the biggest advertising agencies in the country, and embarked on a costly and ambitious advertising campaign in women's magazines and on non-network TV stations. The magazine ads were unusually straightforward for a menstrual product: They used terms like "uterus" and "menstrual flow" instead of euphemisms, and they offered an uncommon money-back guarantee to tempt wary customers. The television ads were equally informational, and they helped drive the wedge that lifted the ban on menstrual product advertising in late 1972.

But the exposure cut two ways. Just as the Tassaway executives were preparing to open an East Coast manufacturing plant, they learned that all of their profits—some $3 million—had been sucked into advertising. With no capital remaining for expansion, plans had to be scrapped. The company never recovered. By late 1972, Tassaway folded its California operation and went out of business.

Before it did, though, it had made millions of converts. In fact, in the late seventies a former Tassaway consultant visited the company's warehouse in Southern California, where he found cartons stamped with dates. Inside the cartons were 20,000 letters from Tassaway customers, and they all said essentially the same thing: "I've been using Tassaway and I love it. Lately, though, it's been increasingly hard to find. Can you help?"

What did women like about Tassaway? Those I've spoken with mention the fact that they were actually able to see their menstrual fluid—and measure how much they'd lost. (They were generally surprised at how small the loss was.) Others had discovered that the "flushable" Tassaway could in fact be reused many times, and they enjoyed the considerable savings that represented. One woman, who had received samples of Tassaway in the doctor's office where she worked, had another interesting observation about the cup. "I've been plagued with vaginal infections all my life," she said. "The only time I didn't have infections is when I used Tassaway."

The menstrual cup has yet another advantage: it can be used to hold medication for the treatment of vaginal infections. It's also been used to collect menstrual fluid in order to diagnose genital tuberculosis (a rare condition) and cancer of the reproductive organs. Dr. Nancy Reame, a reproductive physiologist at the University of Michigan, is using Tassaway cups to study the pH and contents of menstrual fluid.

Some former Tassaway executives held onto the patents and molds and machinery involved in making the cups. During the toxic shock syndrome controversy in 1980, they decided the time was ripe for a comeback. At this writing, they had received the green light from the Food and Drug Administration, had located a production site and were planning to have Tassaway in distribution again sometime in 1981.

Menstrual extraction

Menstrual extraction—the removal of the entire menstrual flow in a simple procedure that lasts about 15 minutes—is not in the strict sense an "alternative" to tampons. It is, instead, a woman-invented, woman-controlled technology that permits, among other things, very early abortion. I include it here because its implications certainly include freedom from the menstrual products industry. I want to emphasize that it is one of the few menstrual alternatives that I have not personally tried. And there have been no controlled, long-term, medically backed studies of its use.

Menstrual extraction was developed in 1972 by Carol Downer, Lorraine Rothman and other women of the Los Angeles Feminist Women's Health Center. Its major stated purpose was to eliminate the "general nuisance" of menstruation and to relieve menstrual symptoms such as cramps, but it was also acknowledged as an important tool for women to learn more about their bodies. Not least, it is a method of birth control by early abortion.

The procedure, as developed by the Los Angeles Feminist Women's Health Center, is always done in small groups, and is usually sponsored by a feminist health clinic. Equipment consists of a Mason jar closed with a rubber stopper, out of which extends two plastic tubes, one of which is connected to a plastic syringe; this apparatus was dubbed the "Del-Em" by its creator, Lorraine Rothman. A valve on the syringe prevents air from being injected into the uterus (a very serious occurrence that could result in death).

The second tube is attached to a very thin (4-millimeter), flexible, sterile piece of tubing called a cannula. The cannula is inserted through the cervical opening (os) by one of the women in the group (not the woman who is having her menses extracted—although she may watch the procedure by using a speculum, a flashlight and a mirror), and draws up the menstrual fluid into the Mason jar.[8,9]

Menstrual extraction has been surrounded by controversy since it was developed. Carelessly practiced, it could cause infection or damage to the uterus. And many doctors feel it would be a very dangerous procedure for a woman whose period was more than two weeks late because of the possibility of its resulting in an incomplete abortion.

Menstrual extraction is probably not something most women would want to do every month. For some women, it's a way of avoiding menstruation if they're prone to very heavy cramps. For others, it's a way of mastering a "medical" technique and breaking down the medical mystique.

Dr. Karnaky's magic bullet

Certainly one of the most bizarre footnotes in the history of menstrual products is the powder-and-tablet technique. More alchemy than "hygiene," it didn't simply absorb or collect the menstrual flow—it transformed it.

This amazing procedure was invented by Dr. Karl John Karnaky, familiar by now as a fan of both tampons and menstrual cups, while he was between enthusiasms. Apparently, the quest for the perfect menstrual product had become something of an obsession with him, as evidenced by his opening statement in a 1959 report on his new method:

> For many years, man has been seeking ways to absorb the menstrual flow during a woman's menstruation, so that during this period she could live her normal life.

Tampons were better than external pads, Karnaky allowed, but not much better: "The absorbed menstrual blood was always loaded with many kinds and shapes of pathogenic and non-pathogenic vaginal microorganisms." Not only that, the tampon's withdrawal string "is almost always found in the area between the buttocks and extending to the anus. Here the string is contaminated with fecal matter and more microorganisms which also contaminate the vaginal canal. . . . The user also contaminates her hand with the bacteria that are on this string."

Thanks to Karnaky's "Menstrual Disorder Clinic," there was good news for us poor bleeders.

With the above in mind, and after seeing thousands of women during their menstrual flow with menstrual blood running down their legs and thighs, all over their perineum and even on their underclothing, this investigator set out to try to find out something that might be labeled at least a small advancement in the handling of menstrual blood.

Karnaky's "advancement" was a combination of powder and tablets. When both were inserted into the vagina just before or during menstruation, they changed menstrual fluid into a "fine, dry, non-sticky, inert, non-toxic sterile powder," highly acidic, which was "apparently" metabolized and reabsorbed into the circulation. The major advantage of this method, Karnaky wrote, was that it circumvented the problem of "deterioration" of menstrual blood, with its accompanying malodors and flourishing bacterial growth.

Karnaky showed 200 women how to use this method (it helped to have some advance warning that one's period was about to begin), but he presented no data on their experiences. He did, however, offer two addresses for physicians wishing to order glass or plastic vaginal powder applicators.[10]

Home remedies

Women made their own tampons at home long before commercial tampons were available, and some women still prefer the do-it-yourself approach. There are several advantages to homemade tampons: They're less expensive than "ready-made," you can be more certain of their contents, and it's easy to make small adjustments in size.

One British woman in her thirties told me that her mother had shown her how to roll tampons out of sterile surgical cotton. "I cut it to size, roll it tightly and insert it," she said. "There's no need for a string—I'm surprised women would want one." She disposes of her tampons in a garbage pail.

The homemade tampon may be more popular in Europe than it is in the United States if the following is an indication. A woman told me of standing in line in a New York restaurant when her period suddenly started. "To my surprise, about ten Frenchwomen standing nearby overheard me mention it to my friends, and they came over and told me about making my own tampons out of gauze." Homemade tampons are now the only menstrual product this woman and her three teenage daughters use.

Another woman reported to me that she swears by cotton balls, which she's used for about five years. "You have to make sure they're cotton—not those rayon 'cosmetic puffs,'" she cautioned. She uses two or three at a time, depending on the amount of her flow, and inserts and removes them with her fingers. "It's clean, cheap and biodegradable," she said. "I also like being involved with my blood—seeing it and feeling it. And it's satisfying to know I exist outside the marketplace of 'feminine' products."

The last word

This story about the ultimate alternative to tampons comes to me courtesy of Emily Culpepper, who has been researching menstrual rituals for eight years. Emily once met a woman who claimed she didn't need *any* menstrual product. Her reason? She had such good control over her vaginal muscles that she could voluntarily retain her menstrual fluid and expel it only when it was convenient.

I'm still practicing.

NOTES

1. Walter G. Larsen, "Sanitary Napkin Dermatitis Due to the Perfume," *Archives of Dermatology* 115 (March 1979):363.

2. Jeannine Parvati, *Hygieia: A Woman's Herbal*, Berkeley, Freestone Collective 1978, p. 15.

3. Alicia Bay Laurel, *Living on the Earth*, Berkeley: Bookworks, 1970 p. 178.

4. Rebecca Liswood, "Internal Menstrual Protection," *Obstetrics and Gynecology*, 13 (May 1959):539.

5. Karnaky, "Internal Menstrual Protection With the Rubber Menstrual Cup," *Obstetrics and Gynecology*, 19 (May 1962):688.

6. Eduardo F. Peña, "Menstrual Protection," *Obstetrics and Gynecology*, 19 (May 1962): 684.

7. John Parker, Robert W. Bushell and S. J. Behrman, "Hygienic Control of Menorrhagia; Use of Rubber Menstrual Cup," *International Journal of Fertility*, 9 (November–December 1964): 619.

8. Lorraine Rothman, "Menstrual Extraction: Procedures," *Quest*, 4 (Summer 1978): 44.

9. Laura Punnett, "Menstrual Extraction: Politics," *Quest*, 4 (Summer 1978): 48.

10. Karnaky, "A New Absorptive for Menstrual Hygiene," *Arizona Medicine*, 16 (September 1959): 605.

CHAPTER 8

Tampons and You

It was at the height of the publicity about toxic shock syndrome. A group of women were talking about tampons, and the more they talked, the angrier they got. "We don't even know what's *in* tampons," one of them exploded. "We've been using them forever, but we still have no idea what they can do to our bodies!"

A male friend happened to pass by and couldn't help overhearing. He was puzzled and bemused. "I realize this has nothing to do with me," he said mildly, "but if you're so upset about tampons, why don't you just stop using them?"

The women looked at each other in surprise. Give up tampons? It was like asking women to give up the vote. Tampons meant freedom: freedom to swim, to go horseback riding, to be a fully active member of society every day of the month . . . just like the ads said. "In recent years women have been making strides in learning to be comfortable with their bodies," one woman reminded me in a letter. "But if our young women are frightened into spending 20 to 25 percent of their time wearing napkins to absorb their menstrual flow, how much of that comfort will remain?" She concluded: "I'll keep my tampons. And my bicycle, running shoes, tennis racket..."

To this woman, tampons are simply another piece of equipment to keep her comfortable and active. But other women question just what sort of "freedom" they're buying each month. Emily Culpepper, whose short film *Period Piece*[1] deals candidly with menstrual ritual and attitudes toward menstruation, calls it "pseudo-liberation." "Tampons are more than a convenience," she says. "They're a way to *hide* our periods. We don't live in the age of the menstrual hut, when women were segregated during their periods so that the rest of the society wouldn't be contaminated. Our menstrual hut is internal, in our heads, so we hide our menses. Look at all the tampon ads that show women wearing white. The implication is that 'no one will know.' Well, maybe it's not so important that no one know."

Even in 1981, that's a radical statement. Somehow we haven't really lost our heritage of the menstrual taboo. Menstruation is still connected with "dirtiness" and disease in some way we don't quite understand, and tampons are our method of exorcising it. "It's an internal/external conflict," Culpepper notes. "If you use an external menstrual product you have to *deal with the blood* in a very different way than if you use tampons." In a culture where blood shed in violence is more acceptable than blood shed during a normal body function, hiding menses has become an obsession—and a profitable one at that.

Toxic shock syndrome served to heighten these underlying fears and guilts about menstruation. After all our attempts to liberate ourselves from the notion that menstruation was a sickness, here were women getting ill and even dying during their periods. Some people thought that TSS was less ominous itself than the emphasis on the association of disease with tampons. As a member of the Berkeley Women's Health Collective told me: "It's as though the government were saying, 'Women have gotten uppity—let's put them back in the home and restrict them with sanitary pads.'"

Many women I talked to about tampons, especially in relation to TSS, felt a sense of betrayal. It wasn't hard to understand. In the United States, menstrual products are advertised like insurance policies: You're not buying merely tampons, you're buying "trust," "confidence" and "protection." Rely "even absorbs the worry." Tampax "takes care of you"—even when you wear white. "I don't worry about tampon accidents," boasts the "liberated" model in the Playtex ad, fist clenched in emphasis. "I say: *Make mine a double!*" (She doesn't mean two tampons, she means Playtex's "double-layered protection.") Toxic shock syndrome—the ultimate "tampon accident"—exposed the menstrual insurance policy as unreliable.

But toxic shock syndrome did more than that. It got us to start talking openly about menstruation and menstrual products—on TV talk shows, on the front pages of newspapers, at home with friends, husbands and lovers. It was a relief to be able to share feelings and ask questions about a subject that had always been shrouded in ignorance and doubt.

The new frankness about menstruation and menstrual products has nothing to do with advertising slogans or raunchy jokes. It has a great deal to do with genuine concern about women's bodies and women's choices. And it's stimulating us to look at tampons in a new way—not as cure-alls, not as poison, but as an option to be approached responsibly, with care and common sense.

If You Choose Tampons

Sandra Ritz, a registered nurse-practitioner, is a women's health editor of *Medical Self-Care* magazine. When TSS hit the news, she was enrolled in a public health graduate program at the University of Hawaii. She'd read about some of the other health problems associated with tampons—ulcerations, lacerations, reactions to the fragrance in "deodorant" tampons. And by asking around she learned that most women—especially younger women—were easily influenced when it came to buying tampons. "Older women tend to buy whatever tampon is on sale," she notes. "Younger women are much more susceptible to advertising." At the same time, most of the women she talked to seemed to have little knowledge about what tampons actually were, and how they worked.

Ritz decided that what was needed was some solid information about tampons and TSS—not a sales pitch or a scare tactic. She prepared a one-hour presentation about tampons for a mixed class—boys and girls—of juniors and seniors at a Honolulu high school. (She is now working on an informational videotape about tampons and toxic shock syndrome.)

"I start with very basic information," Ritz explains. "I ask, What is a tampon? What motivates you to buy them? Then I say that maybe we need to realize that tampons are a medical device, not just something you buy to make you popular or because you want to wear white."

Ritz's advice about tampon use makes sense for women of all ages, not just teenagers. Here are some of the things she suggests:

• *Look at tampons.*
Take them apart. Cut them open. Observe them after they've been dunked in water. ("Some brands leave particles in the water," says Ritz.) See whether they expand lengthwise or through their width. "A virgin might be more comfortable with a tampon that expands lengthwise," Ritz says, "while a woman who's had one or more vaginal childbirth deliveries might prefer a tampon that expands sideways."

• *Choose a tampon that's only as absorbent as you need.*

"Some tampons are so absorbent that they dry the vagina, absorbing its normal secretions. Think of the dentist's cotton and how it feels when you have to keep it in your mouth. A too-absorbent tampon can have the same effect." Ritz adds that since women's flows vary over the course of a single menstrual period, it's a good idea to keep tampons of different absorbencies for heavy and light days. If your vagina seems dry when you remove a tampon, switch to a less-absorbent tampon—or to a mini-pad or panty liner.

• *Be wary of "deodorant" tampons*.

"The only thing they deodorize is the garbage can or the toilet. Be aware of allergic reactions like burning, itching or discharge. Remember, menstrual blood has no odor until it reaches the air."

• *Try going without tampons for one menstrual period*.

"See whether it makes a difference. You may discover that tampons had been irritating, or that a chronic infection clears up. On the other hand, you may find that pads are too much of a bother. And in some women, pads contribute to bladder infections. Experiment a little—but be aware you're experimenting."

• *Change tampons every 4 to 6 hours, depending on need*.

"For example, if the flow is heavy, change every 2 to 4 hours; if it's moderate, every 4 to 5 hours; and if it's light, every 5 to 6 hours. This will vary with each woman. You just have to experiment. But don't wear the same tampon all day and all night—that encourages bacteria to grow in the vagina's dark moist climate. On the other hand, don't change every half hour—that can be very irritating."

• *Always remove the last tampon you insert*.

"It sounds obvious, but I've talked to many women who say they've left tampons in their vaginas for more than 24 hours. They probably aren't risking anything more than a bad-smelling discharge, but it's a matter of becoming more aware of your body. A tampon isn't lipstick or face cream—it's something you put in the interior of your body."

• *Don't use tampons when you're not menstruating*.

"In a study I did recently, nearly a fifth of the women I surveyed said they used tampons for reasons other than menstruation—for example, because they didn't want to wear underpants. When you're not menstruating, a tampon absorbs your normal vaginal lubrication, which is there to protect you from infection." Recent research has also shown that women who wear tampons for extended periods of time have an increased chance of developing ulcerations of the vagina.

- *Trust your intuition.*

"A lot of women have TSS symptoms but don't tell their doctors because they're afraid they won't be taken seriously. If you have any kind of medical problem, tune into your body and make connections. A good way to do this is to keep a diary."

- *Become an informed consumer.*

"Yes, you *can* use tampons—it's unrealistic to say you can't. But you are at the mercy of big business—so make sure your choice is an educated one."

The Future of Tampons

I knew from dozens of conversations and interviews that many women were dissatisfied with the menstrual products available to them. And I knew that, for some women, the reason for the dissatisfaction was the sense that an industry dominated by men couldn't answer women's needs. So I asked women to pretend *they* were in control. I posed the question: If you could design the "ideal" menstrual product, what would it be?

Many women thought commercial tampons could be improved—for starters by making them less expensive. There seemed to be an undercurrent of resentment that women had to pay a premium for a product they needed for a normal body function.

"Safe" and "biodegradable" were mentioned almost as often. "Plastic applicators are hard to dispose of," one woman complained. However, another woman liked "the smoothness of the plastic applicator. It doesn't pinch." Couldn't a smooth yet biodegradable material be developed? A third women pointed out that *all* tampons presented a disposal problem. I'm sure plumbers would agree with her: Although tampons are promoted as flushable, they take a long time to decay. In the meantime they balloon in the pipes, wreaking havoc.

Some other comments about "ideal" tampons:

—"Need more variation in absorbency."
—"More assurance about actual material used."
—"Would like to be assured product is sterile and made of safe material like cotton, not synthetics or abrasives."
—"No unnecessary applicators or packing, please."
—"Safe and cheap . . . comfortable applicator."

Several women said they'd already found the ideal menstrual product in the sea sponge. "I have used sea sponges for over three years," one woman wrote. "One of these lasted at least a year before it began to tear. I have never had any problems—no infections, no irritation or drying of my vagina. I once used one that was too large (pressure on my bladder), so I cut it down in size. Women could spend a dollar or less a year for their periods."

Another sponge fan wrote, "I love having no string. Always hated the string on tampons—never felt really naked."

Other women thought the sponge could be improved. "I'd like to see sponges grown under controlled conditions and bred for absorbency," wrote one. Another favored disposable sponges for use during vaginal infections, reusable ones for menstruation.

A few women put their imaginations to work creating totally new menstrual products. "An absorbent panty could be invented, one that would absorb a full day's flow without any suggestion of odor or blood," one woman recommended. "The panty could be laundered and used again whenever the woman was menstruating. Women would probably own several 'tampanties' just as they own bras and regular, everyday panties. I have yet to figure out the remarkable new absorbent material that would be used to create these 'tampanties,' but I'm working on it."

Another woman suggested "a little rag made out of a leaf with a sticky substance to attach to underpants. It would come in a variety of shapes that corresponded to one's flow. It would be free for all women except for the costs of gathering, shaping and distributing. If we can fly to the moon, we should be able to figure *this* out."

Finally, one woman proposed a reusable menstrual cup made of plastic or latex. "Flexible tabs for insertion would help," she added. This "future menstrual product" is actually an old idea—the Tassette rubber menstrual cup was first marketed in the early fifties. It was updated in the late sixties by the Tassaway company, which developed a patented plastic material that softened when it came into contact with body heat. And now it's being revived: A Tassaway spokesman predicted that menstrual cups would be available again by mid-1981. Unfortunately, the plastic cups have a much shorter life span than the original rubber: They can be used four or five times, but begin to lose their shape soon afterward.

Beyond Tampons

As consumers, women have the power—and the responsibility—to make changes in the menstrual products industry. If we don't like the way tampons are made or marketed, we can let their manufacturers know, either by writing letters or by boycotting products we object to.

But that's only a first step. The tampon issue has implications that go beyond tampons themselves. To start at the source, we now know that our store of information about menstruation is woefully inadequate. We don't know enough about amount of flow, contents of menstrual fluid, or what causes cramps—and all of these areas bear directly on the design of menstrual products. For example, if we knew more about what was in menstrual fluid, and in what proportions, tampon makers might be able to test absorbency with a more reliable substance than saline or gelatin solutions.

We need to expand our knowledge about normal body functions *in general*. Not just menstruation but aging, menopause, pregnancy and childbirth need to be reexamined as states of health, not disease.

And while re-examining these normal body functions we ought to consider more seriously the commercial products related to them. For example, the newest diapers on the market use the same superabsorbent fibers that tampons do. Some of them are designed to fit a baby's bottom so snugly that no moisture can possibly escape. That's great for the baby's parents—but what about the baby? Does the sealed-off diaper become a trap for multiplying bacteria? By the way, the problem isn't limited to babies—there are super-absorbent diapers for incontinent adults (the elderly, the ill, the mentally retarded) as well.

Other products that come into intimate contact with the body have also been overlooked for too long. Nearly all contraceptive jellies, foams and creams contain perfume. Is it really necessary? Can it cause allergic reactions? What about the lubricant on condoms—how can we know what it's made of? Do fabric softeners and scented toilet paper play a role in chronic itching?

"The lesson to be learned from this tampon market problem," wrote a stock brokerage analyst in the fall of 1980, "is that regardless of how thoroughly a company test-markets its product and how successful it eventually becomes in the actual marketplace, a medical or health care product can directly or indirectly cause serious adverse reactions, resulting in FDA action to protect the consumer."[2]

That was written from the corporate point of view, as a way of warning companies that their best efforts may not be good enough. But it serves as a warning to consumers too. As we learn to accept our bodies and their cycles, we need to learn to question the companies that ask us to entrust our bodies to them. We need to know what substances we're inserting into our bodies. We need to know the risks we take when we insert those substances. We need to ask questions, and we have a right to expect honest answers.

But more than just being good consumers, we need to begin taking control of the consumables—the products and services—aimed at women. The women's self-care movement is an excellent example of the kind of system that can evolve when women actively participate in their own health needs. But the self-care movement isn't enough. More women need to go beyond it—into basic research, into epidemiology, into public health—so that the fundamental questions so important to women are asked.

Finally, we need to make the menstrual products industry a *women's* industry. On a very small scale, that's already happening: Sea sponge distributors have been mostly female, and in California, reusable menstrual pads are being produced by woman-owned, woman-controlled companies. More are needed, with more women setting the priorities and choosing the materials. Tampons and other menstrual products are women's concern: It's time to make them women's business as well.

NOTES

1. "Period Piece," a 10-minute 16-millimeter color film, is available for sale or rent through Emily Culpepper, 1116 East 33rd St., Oakland, California, 94610.

2. From Neil B. Sweig, "Problems in the U.S. Tampon Market," prepared for Shearson Loeb Rhoades Inc., September 29, 1980.

Appendix

Where to write or phone if you have questions about tampons or other menstrual products.

1. Manufacturers

ASSURE! (currently in test market only)
  Arlene C. Krupinski
  Director, Consumer Affairs
  Personal Products Company
  Milltown, New Jersey 08850
  201 524–7852

KOTEX (stick and tube tampons)
  Ron Goudreau
  Director, Public Relations Services

  Dr. Eugene R. Jolly
  Director, Product Safety
  Kimberly-Clark Corporation
  Neenah, Wisconsin 54956
  414 721–2000

O.B.

Jane H. Yates
Vice President, Consumer Affairs
Johnson & Johnson Products, Inc.
501 George Street
New Brunswick, New Jersey 08903
201 524–0400

o.b. Information Center (toll-free)
800 526–2433 (in New Jersey, 800 352–4777)
Call on business days between 10 a.m. and 4 p.m.,
Eastern time

PLAYTEX

Leonard Berger
Director, Consumer Affairs
International Playtex, Inc.
Box 728
Paramus, New Jersey 07652
201 265–8000

PURSETTES

Eldon Miller
Vice President, Corporate Relations
Campana Corporation
Division of Purex Industries
5101 Clark Avenue
Lakewood, California 90712
213 634–3300

TAMPAX

Dr. Clayton L. Thomas
Vice President, Medical Affairs
Tampax Incorporated
Box 271
Palmer, Massachusetts 01069
413 283–3434

Vera J. Milow
Vice President, Educational Affairs
Tampax Incorporated
Lake Success, New York 11042
516 437–8800

TASSAWAY (menstrual cup)
Shirley Squire
Representative
Tassaway, Inc.
108 East Hillcrest Road
Orlando, Florida 32801
305 841–8010

2. Consumer organizations

HEALTH RESEARCH GROUP
Dr. Sidney Wolfe
Director
2000 P Street N.W.
Washington, D.C. 20036
202 872–0320

NATIONAL WOMEN'S HEALTH NETWORK
Elayne Clift
Network Program Director
224 7th Street S.E.
Washington, D.C. 20003
202 543–9222

3. Government agencies

CENTERS FOR DISEASE CONTROL
  Bob Alden
  Public information
  Atlanta, Georgia 30333
  404 329–3286

FOOD AND DRUG ADMINISTRATION

The FDA has district offices in the following cities: Atlanta, Baltimore, Boston, Buffalo, Chicago, Dallas, Denver, Detroit, Kansas City, Los Angeles, Minneapolis, Nashville, Newark, New Orleans, New York, Orlando, Philadelphia, San Francisco, San Juan (Puerto Rico) and Seattle. You may file a complaint about tampons or other medical devices through the district office nearest your home.

Or you may file directly into the

DEVICE EXPERIENCE NETWORK
8757 Georgia Avenue, Room 1222
HFK-125
Silver Spring, Maryland
202 427–8100

ABOUT THE AUTHOR

Nancy Friedman was born in Los Angeles in 1950, attended Los Angeles public schools and was graduated from the University of California at Berkeley. She is a former editor of *New West* magazine, and has published many articles about women's issues. "The Truth About Tampons," her investigative article about tampon hazards for *New West*, was a 1980 finalist for the National Magazine Award and the Sigma Delta Chi (journalism society) award. She lives in Berkeley, California.

index

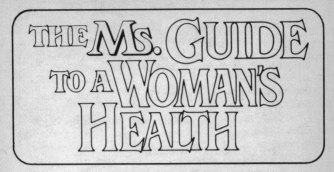